NON-DRUG TREATMENTS FOR ESSENTIAL HYPERTENSION

Pergamon Titles of Related Interest

Belar/Deardorff/Kelly/ THE PRACTICE OF CLINICAL HEALTH
PSYCHOLOGY

Blanchard/Andrasik/ MANAGEMENT OF CHRONIC HEADACHES:
A Psychological Approach

Blechman/Brownell/ HANDBOOK OF BEHAVIORAL MEDICINE
FOR WOMEN

Holzman/Turk/ PAIN MANAGEMENT: A Handbook of Psychological
Treatment Approaches

Russell/ STRESS MANAGEMENT FOR CHRONIC DISEASE

Related Journals*

CLINICAL PSYCHOLOGY REVIEW

JOURNAL OF PSYCHOSOMATIC RESEARCH

SOCIAL SCIENCE AND MEDICINE

*Free sample copies available upon request

PSYCHOLOGY PRACTITIONER GUIDEBOOKS

EDITORS
Arnold P. Goldstein, Syracuse University
Leonard Krasner, Stanford University & SUNY at Stony Brook
Sol L. Garfield, Washington University in St. Louis

NON-DRUG TREATMENTS FOR ESSENTIAL HYPERTENSION

EDWARD B. BLANCHARD
State University of New York at Albany

JOHN E. MARTIN
San Diego State University & University of California,
San Diego, Medical School

PATRICIA M. DUBBERT
Jackson Veterans Administration Medical Center
and University of Mississippi Medical Center

PERGAMON PRESS
New York · Oxford · Beijing · Frankfurt
São Paulo · Sydney · Tokyo · Toronto

U.S.A.	Pergamon Press, Inc., Maxwell House, Fairview Park, Elmsford, New York 10523, U.S.A.
U.K	Pergamon Press plc, Headington Hill Hall, Oxford OX3 0BW, England
PEOPLE'S REPUBLIC OF CHINA	Pergamon Press, Room 4037, Qianmen Hotel, Beijing, People's Republic of China
FEDERAL REPUBLIC OF GERMANY	Pergamon Press GmbH, Hammerweg 6, D-6242 Kronberg, Federal Republic of Germany
BRAZIL	Pergamon Editora Ltda, Rua Eça de Queiros, 346, CEP 04011, Paraiso, São Paulo, Brazil
AUSTRALIA	Pergamon Press Australia Pty Ltd., P.O. Box 544, Potts Point, N.S.W. 2011, Australia
JAPAN	Pergamon Press, 5th Floor, Matsuoka Central Building, 1-7-1 Nishishinjuku, Shinjuku-ku, Tokyo 160, Japan
CANADA	Pergamon Press Canada Ltd., Suite No. 271, 253 College Street, Toronto, Ontario, Canada M5T 1R5

First edition 1988

Library of Congress Cataloging in Publication Data

Blanchard, Edward B.
Non-drug treatments for essential hypertension /
Edward B. Blanchard, John E. Martin, Patricia Dubbert :
with a foreword by Herbert G. Langford.
p. cm. — (Psychology practitioner guidebooks)
Bibliography: p.
Includes index.
1. Hypertension—Treatment. 2. Hypertension—Diet
therapy. 3. Exercise therapy.
4. Hypertension—Psychosomatic aspects.
5. Stress (Psychology) I. Martin, John E.
1947–   . II. Dubbert, Patricia M. III. Title.
IV. Series.
[DNLM 1. Hypertension—therapy. WG 340 B639n]
RC685.H8B59   1988
616.1'3206—dc19   87-25844 CIP

British Library Cataloguing in Publication Data

Blanchard, Edward B.
Non-drug treatments for essential
hypertension.—(Psychology practitioner
guidebooks).
1. Hyperlipidemia—Diet therapy
I. Title II. Martin, John E. III. Dubbert
Patricia IV. Series
616.3'9970654   RC632.H87

ISBN 0-08-032809-1 Hard cover
ISBN 0-08-032808-3 Flexicover

Printed in Great Britain by A. Wheaton & Co. Ltd., Exeter

Dedication

To my mentors in this area and others, Albert Bandura, Henry Adams, and Stewart Agras. (EBB)

To one who has devoted his entire research career to the understanding of hypertension, and who has so greatly influenced us all, Arthur Guyton; and to the Master who has so graciously given us the tools of Science and Truth. May this bear fruit for any in need. (JEM)

To Randy, Robert, and Douglas with love. (PMD)

Contents

Acknowledgments

All three of us owe a great intellectual and personal debt to Dr. Herbert G. Langford for his gentle tutelage and professional support as we learned about hypertension and its treatment.

I would like to acknowledge the support of the National Heart, Lung and Blood Institute, through grants HL–14906, HL–18814, HL–27622, and HL–31189, over the period 1972 through 1987, for supporting much of my research in hypertension. I would also like to acknowledge collaborators and colleagues over this interval: Larry D. Young, Mary Ruth Haynes, Gene G. Abel, Rebecca Wicker, Steve Miller, William Murphy, Guy C. McCoy, Robert McCaffrey, and Frank Andrasik. I also want to thank the graduate students at SUNY-Albany who assisted in this research: Tom Pallmeyer, Rob Gerardi, Maryrose A. Gerardi, Pat Guarnieri, Mindy Halpern, Alison Musso, David Wittrock, Marta Berger, and Cynthia Radnitz. Finally, I would like to express appreciation to Sandy Agosto for preparing the many parts and versions of this manuscript. (EBB)

I would like to acknowledge the support of the Medical Research Service of the Veterans Administration, through grant IIR81–62 of the Health Services Research and Development, for supporting the bulk of my research in hypertension. William C. Cushman served as co-investigator of the main hypertension project and was instrumental in the planning, conducting and analyzing of our hypertension studies. In addition, I want to thank Leonard H. Epstein, Neil B. Oldridge, and Herbert G. Langford for serving as consultants during the planning and course of the project, and Edward Meydrech and Robert Carroll, who helped conduct statistical and biochemical analyses. Technical support for the projects was ably provided by Mary Elizabeth Lake and Paul Anthony Burkett. Thanks are extended to James G. Hollandsworth and Rebecca Martin for their critical reading of portions of this book, and to Nancy (Mary) Yonkers and Ann Walker for their tireless technical work and typing on sections of the manuscript. Colleagues who influenced me importantly during my Mississippi years include Leonard H. Epstein, Lee W. Frederiksen, Patricia M. Dubbert, James G. Hollandsworth, Terence M. Keane, Donald M. Prue, William G. Johnson, Jeffery S. Webster, and Ellie T. Sturgis. A very special thanks is extended to my invaluable clinical research associate and good friend Bill Richter, without whose support, humor, and exceptional hard work many of our clinical research programs would not have been nearly so successful. The role of Pat Dubbert in the behavioral hypertension research that stemmed from our program is incalculable—she has been a colleague extraordinaire, excellent co-author, and friend over the years. Finally, appreciation is expressed to the following, who as clinical psychology residents (interns) made valuable contributions to our hypertension research and treatment programs: Tim Ahles, John Arena, Robert Brubaker, Randye Cohen, Patricia Cole, Frank Collins, Sheila Corrigan, Leonard Doerfler, Jeffrey Dolce, Maria Ekstrand, Michael Faulstich, James Fitterling, Joel Haber, Janel Harris, Danny Kaloupek, Alan Katell, Abby King, Thomas Lombardo, Joanie Mayer, Eric Morrell, Charles Morin, Deborah Ossip-Klein, Thomas Payne, Kenneth Perkins, James Raczynski, Steven Rapp, Neil Rappaport, David Schlundt, Kevin Thompson, Marilyn Zegman, and Rose Zimering. (JEM)

I am indebted to many individuals for their encouragement and collaboration in my research in behavioral medicine. Special acknowledgment is due to G. Terence Wilson, John E. Martin, and Terence Keane for their guidance in graduate school, residency training, and beyond; and to my colleagues and the University of Mississippi–Jackson Veterans Administration Medical Center psychology residents who contributed to the success of the Heart Health Program. (PMD)

Foreword

There is overwhelming epidemiological evidence that blood pressure is significantly correlated with body weight and sodium intake. However, increased intake of potassium, calcium, magnesium, and unsaturated fats may affect the blood pressure level by blocking the blood pressure-raising effects of sodium. In addition, evidence mounts that increased aerobic exercise can also decrease blood pressure, and that there are, at least, short-term benefits from relaxation and similar forms of therapy.

The central focus of this monograph is that it is now possible to induce behavioral change to allow weight loss, increased exercise, and the other desirable modifications noted above. For years, I have suggested to my patients that they lose weight. The usual response has been modest weight gain. Many physicians—in the past I have been among them—feel that they do better with changing sodium intake than changing weight. However, physicians rarely measure sodium excretion; therefore, the physician and perhaps the patient will feel that the results of the physician's admonitions are appreciably better than the facts warrant. Similarly, my admonition to increase exercise produces, I would estimate, about $3\frac{1}{2}$-hour walks. That figure is based on my "successful" patients. The chapters in this volume well document that behavior change programs run by skilled professionals have a vastly better record than the one I described.

As it is now possible to induce relatively long-lasting behavioral change, where shall this modality be applied? Which patients will benefit? Which patients can use behavioral change as a substitute for medication?

A consideration of the factors entering into the attained pressure exhibited by the patient can give guidance as to the applicability of behavioral change at various points in the patient's history. We can consider the attained pressure as a consequence of: (a) heredity; (b) environmental forces (obesity, electrolyte intake, perhaps intake of saturated fats, and psychological factors); and finally (c) hypertrophy of the arterioles—a perpetuating or perhaps even multiplicative factor, as described by Folkow. Hypertrophy of the arterioles occurs as a result of hypertension. The hypertrophied arteriole responds more enthusiastically to vasoconstrictor stimuli than the non-hypertrophied arteriole. Therefore, a less pronounced stimulus than was required for producing hypertension may be adequate to continue and perpetuate the hypertension.

Let us take a hypothetical example involving sodium. Many investigators feel that we should take less than 70 meq of sodium daily. A male patient has been ingesting 200 meq of sodium daily and has become definitely hypertensive. If, prior to onset, his diet had contained only 100 meq of sodium, he probably would not have developed elevated blood pressure. Now that he has hypertrophied arterioles, reduction to 100 meq sodium daily is inadequate to restore him to normotension. Pharmacological therapy will be necessary, at least for a time.

With this principle in mind, I wish to interpret the published material on behavioral change and blood pressure. Incidentally, when making scientific decisions in this field, one should use only studies which have been fully randomized; if possible, the person measuring blood pressure should have been blind to the therapy being used. Unfortunately, we find an amazing paucity of such well-conducted studies demonstrating the benefit of behavioral change as sole therapy, especially if we also insist that the studies have followed the participants at least half a year. MacMahon's study of the effect of weight loss in obese hypertensives is one of the few exceptions. The randomized participants lost an average of 15 pounds, with a very satisfactory drop in blood pressure compared both to their base line pressures and to the control group. Another study by Logan found no benefit from 5 pounds weight loss. The situation for other modalities is even less well documented.

The situation is different when we look at the effect of weight change and change in sodium intake in the treated hypertensive patient. Reisin's paper remains an important mile post. Relatively severe hypertensive patients randomized to weight loss had a significant drop in blood pressure and in antihypertensive medication requirement, compared to their colleagues who were not so treated. Other studies show similar benefit for decreased sodium intake.

The incentive for many patients to consider behavioral change is the hope that their hypertension can be managed without any drugs at all.

There are now two studies showing the benefit of weight loss and sodium restriction in the patient in whom drug therapy was stopped after a number of years. I believe that the results are good enough for this approach—that of drug treatment followed or accompanied by behavioral change—to be considered for almost all hypertensive patients. The minority of hypertensive patients who had very severe hypertension, or who required multiple drugs for therapy, probably should not be considered for stopping medication, but they can certainly benefit from weight loss and reduced sodium intake.

On theoretical grounds, the most logical place for behavioral change in the whole problem of hypertension is in its prevention. I sincerely believe that many hypertension-prone individuals could prevent the development of hypertension if they would stay at or close to their lean weights; exercise regularly; keep sodium intake low and potassium intake high; and perhaps handle the normal stress of their lives with equanimity.

There is a major clinical problem requiring behavioral assistance which none of the authors have addressed, except briefly in Chapters 2 and 9. This is the smoking hypertensive patient.

Stopping smoking is the most important move that the patient can make. However, almost all patients gain weight on stopping smoking. Therefore we must design a program that will not only help the patient to stop smoking but will prevent the weight gain that so frequently follows cessation of smoking.

In summary, almost every hypertensive patient needs help with behavioral change. I feel that the best role for behavioral change is first, in combination with drug therapy, and second, to allow continued normotension for some patients after discontinuation of previously successful drug therapy.

Behavioral change approaches as outlined in this volume, used in the right context, are invaluable additions to our armamentarium, and should be used with increasing frequency.

Herbert G. Langford, M.D.
The University of Mississippi Medical Center
2500 North State Street
Jackson, MS 39216

Introduction

This book arose out of our mutual interests in a single topic, non-drug treatments for hypertension. Each of us spent a number of years working as a clinical psychologist and faculty member at the University of Mississippi Medical Center and Jackson VA in Jackson, Mississippi. In those capacities we came under the influence of two of the giants in the field of essential hypertension, Arthur Guyton and Herbert Langford, who supported our interests as behavioral psychologists in their field of hypertension.

Each of us had his or her own sub-field of expertise in the non-drug treatments of hypertension. The interest in the sub-fields, stress management for Blanchard, dietary interventions for Dubbert, and exercise for Martin, arose before the interest in hypertension. However, hypertension provided a fertile field in which our expertise could flourish. The complex, multifactorial nature of essential hypertension demands complex multifactorial treatments, especially among the non-drug treatment approaches. Hence, our collaboration on this book.

This book, as one of the Pergamon Practitioner Guidebooks, is written primarily for the practitioner. It is also written primarily for the non-medical practitioner. However, with the growing interest in the medical community (Brandt, Assistant Secretary for Health, 1983; Joint National Committee, 1986) in non-drug treatments for hypertension, and the general absence of expertise in these approaches among medical personnel, much of the book has relevance for the medical practitioner as well.

In this book we have attempted to do several things. We start by providing basic information on the epidemiology of hypertension and effects of drug treatment on it (Chapter 1). Next is a brief chapter (Chapter 2) to help the reader understand the complex interacting physiological processes which regulate blood pressure. There follows a chapter (Chapter 3) on initial assessment procedures including taking a history, measuring blood pressure and the role of psychological tests.

With this preliminary, but necessary, information out of the way, the next five chapters describe the major non-drug treatments for hypertension. In each of these chapters we have tried to do three things: (1) to provide a brief summary of the literature on the use of the procedure with hypertension; (2) to describe in detail how to implement the particular procedure and (3) to describe our own results with the procedure. Thus, all of the procedures and techniques described in Chapters 4 through 8 have been tested by one of us on hypertensive patients. Thus, Blanchard describes Relaxation (Chapter 4) and Biofeedback (Chapter 5) as Stress Management procedures. Martin describes establishing exercise programs (Chapter 6) while Dubbert describes various dietary approaches (Chapter 7). As a final behavioral intervention we have described in Chapter 8 how to improve antihypertensive medication compliance.

For convenience and clarity, the treatments have been compartmentalized into separate chapters. However, as practitioners, one may need to use all of these procedures in a single patient. The final chapter (Chapter 9) is our attempt to describe how "to put it all together."

We are pleased with the product and hope it is of benefit to you, the practitioner, and to your patients.

Chapter 1

Hypertension: Epidemiology and Medical Treatment

EPIDEMIOLOGY OF ELEVATED BLOOD PRESSURE

Heart and blood vessel diseases have been the major causes of death in the United States for more than 40 years and now account for half of all deaths. More than two Americans suffer heart attacks every minute (Levy & Moskowitz, 1982). Even though deaths due to heart disease have declined by 26% and deaths due to stroke have declined by 48% during the last couple of decades (Haber, 1985), the total cost of cardiovascular disease (CVD) is still estimated to be in excess of $60 billion annually and CVD accounts for more bed days than any other single condition (Levy & Moskowitz, 1982). Many factors have probably contributed to the recent decline in CVD mortality, including improved medical services, the development of coronary care units, advances in surgical and medical treatment, and improved control of blood pressure. Proponents of nondrug treatments, however, are particularly encouraged by evidence that changes in behavioral risk factors such as smoking, leisure-time activities, and eating habits have contributed significantly to these improvements in life expectancy (Haber, 1985).

Epidemiology is the branch of medicine that studies the relationship among various factors that determine frequencies and distributions of a disease. Epidemiologic research has yielded a great deal of information about the numbers and characteristics of individuals who have CVD and about the factors that when present place particular individuals at increased risk for the development and manifestation of these conditions (Pollock, Wilmore, & Fox, 1984). Hypertension, which may affect one out of every three Americans, is the most common CVD and has been consistently identified as a major risk factor for coronary heart disease (Castelli, 1984; Subcommittee on Definition and Prevalence, 1985). Knowledge of risk factors for CVD morbidity (disease frequency) and mortality (deaths) is important in helping clinicians identify populations most in need of intervention and in setting priorities with individual patients.

Factors Associated with Elevated Blood Pressure

Age. Many epidemiologic surveys have shown a general tendency for blood pressure (BP) to rise with age. Normal blood pressure in infants and young children is much lower than in adults. BP rises steeply as the child grows, reaches somewhat of a plateau when adult height is reached, and, in Western societies, typically continues to rise gradually and then more steeply with advancing age (Page, 1983). In the United States, the prevalence of hypertension (defined as blood pressure greater than 140/90 or self-reported taking of antihypertensive medication) is higher in older age groups. This finding is true for blacks, whites, men, and women. In fact, recent survey data indicate that, among persons 55 years of age and older, 50% or more have hypertension (Subcommittee on Definition and Prevalence, 1985).

Heredity. Although the mode of inheritance has yet to be clarified, there is general agreement that heredity is an extremely potent determinant of adult blood pressure (Page, 1983). Studies of the concordance of blood pressure between relatives show that correlation coefficients are highest among monozygotic twins and lower as shared genetic background diminishes. Adoption studies have found the expected correlations between biological parents and children's blood pressures, with no correlation between blood pressures of parents and their adopted children (Biron, Mongeau, & Bertrand, 1976).

Sex. Other things being equal, hypertension is found somewhat more frequently in men (33.0%) than in women (26.8%). During young adulthood, hypertension is more prevalent in men but, after 55 years of age, the rates for women catch up with and then surpass those for men. In part this reflects the higher prevalence of isolated systolic hypertension (SBP greater than 140 mm Hg (mercury) with diastolic [DPB] readings in the normal range) in older women and the longer life expectancy of women (Subcommittee on Definition and Prevalence, 1985).

Race. Elevated blood pressure is much more common in blacks (38.2%) than in whites (28.8%) in the United States (Subcommittee on Definition and Prevalence, 1985). Morbidity and mortality for blacks are also excessive compared with the white population (Prineas & Gillum, 1985). Hypertension also tends to be more severe in blacks, which may be due to the average younger age at onset, greater susceptibility to target organ damage, and/or beginning adequate therapy later. Severe hypertension is four times as frequent in black as compared with white men, while isolated systolic hypertension is more common among older black women. In black women aged 65 to 74 years, the dual risk factors of age and race contribute to the very high prevalence of 82.9% (Subcommittee on Definition and Prevalence, 1985).

Body mass and obesity. Weight gain during adult life is an important risk factor for the development of hypertension, and almost every epidemiologic survey has found significant correlations between blood pressure and body mass, and between hypertension and obesity (Subcommittee on Nonpharmacological Therapy, 1986). In the Framingham study, the group who became 20% or more over ideal weight were eight times more likely to become hypertensive. The mechanisms through which body mass or obesity influence blood pressure are unknown, but the relationship holds true even in populations where sodium intake is low. Loss of weight is often associated with clinically significant decreases in blood pressure, even if the loss is much less than that required for the individual to reach ideal weight (Eliahou, Iaina, Gaon, Shochat, & Modan, 1981). Behavioral interventions to assist the overweight hypertensive in weight reduction will be discussed in detail in Chapter 7.

Dietary electrolyte intake. Although there has been considerable debate about dietary electrolytes, particularly sodium, potassium, and calcium, we still do not understand the role of these variables in the development and treatment of hypertension. A correlation between average daily intake of sodium and frequency of hypertension can be shown at the extremes of very high and very low intake. However, no clear relationship between sodium intake and blood pressure level has been shown within populations, and the extreme high- and low-sodium-intake populations tend to differ on many more variables as well. For example, the less industrialized populations with low sodium intake also tend to have high potassium intakes, do not gain weight with age, and are more active physically. Intervention trials indicate that sodium restriction benefits some but not all hypertensives (Subcommittee on Nonpharmacological Therapy, 1986). Restricted-sodium diets are discussed in Chapter 7 in the section on dietary interventions.

Very-low-sodium diets are almost always high in potassium, so it has been suggested that this is an alternative explanation for the lower prevalence of hypertension in low-sodium-intake populations. At present, relatively little is known about the effects of potassium on normal or hypertensive persons. A few studies of the effects of potassium supplementation in mild hypertensives have now been reported, but the results thus far are variable at best (Subcommittee on Nonpharmacological Therapy, 1986). Epidemiological data on calcium intake and hypertension have also been a recent focus of interest. However, there has been considerable debate about the interpretation of these data and there was insufficient evidence from intervention trials at the time this chapter was written to determine if calcium supplementation has therapeutic value (Subcommittee on Non-pharmacological Therapy, 1986).

Alcohol intake. Although people who report they drink small amounts of alcohol have lower pressures than nondrinkers, several studies have shown a significant relationship between alcohol intake and blood pressure. High alcohol intake now appears to be an important risk factor for hypertension (Page, 1983).

Prevalence and Treatment of Elevated Blood Pressure in the USA

The most recent definitions of hypertension take into account advances in understanding of both blood-pressure-related risks and the efficacy of antihypertensive therapy (Working Group on Risk and High Blood Pressure, 1985). Individuals are now placed in minimal-risk, intermediate-risk, or higher risk categories according to specified systolic and/or diastolic BP readings on the first and second occasion of measurement. Thus, the new definitions also take into account the tendency for readings to be higher at an initial reading in a new situation. Table 1–1 shows the current recommended classification scheme.

According to the new definitions, in the United States alone there are 58 million persons at increased risk of disease and premature death associated with high blood pressure. Although there have been great improvements in the number of persons who are aware of their hypertension and have access to adequate treatment, it is still estimated that only a little more than 50% of hypertensives are aware of their condition and that the number of hypertensives whose blood pressure is adequately controlled is only about 34% (using 160/90 as a cutoff). Control rates are even lower (11%) if a threshold of 140/90 is used. Control rates are especially low for young persons aged 18 to 24 years

Table 1-1. Recommended Classification Scheme for Arterial Blood Pressure in Adults (Joint National Committee on Detection, Evaluation, and Treatment of High Blood Pressure, 1984)

Diastolic Blood Pressure	Category
≤ 85 mm Hg	Normal blood pressure
85 to 89 mm Hg	High normal blood pressure
90 to 104 mm Hg	Mild hypertension
105 to 114 mm Hg	Moderate hypertension
≥ 115 mm Hg	Severe hypertension

Systolic Blood Pressure when diastolic blood pressure is > 90 mm Hg	Category
< 140 mm Hg	Normal blood pressure
140–159 mm Hg	Borderline isolated systolic hypertension
≥ 160 mm Hg	Isolated systolic hypertension

(only 2.2%), and are worse for men (6.1%) than for women (16.7%). It is clear that only a small percent of persons who can benefit from treatment of hypertension have been reached.

WHY SHOULD HYPERTENSION BE TREATED?

In today's health care climate, the title of this section may seem a bit strange, but as little as 20 years ago it was a very legitimate question. In the early 1960s the long-term serious sequelae of hypertension had been known for some time, and it had been established that the treatment of malignant hypertension could be life saving (Dustan et al., 1958; Sokolow & Perloff, 1960; Mohler & Freis, 1960). However, in the early 1960s there was still a debate in the medical community over whether essential hypertension should be treated and especially whether successful lowering of BP made any significant difference in morbidity or mortality (Perera, 1960; Goldring & Chasis, 1965; Relman, 1966).

1967 VA Cooperative Study

The first definitive answer to the latter question, that is, one based on a randomized clinical trial, was conducted by the Veterans Administration (VA) Cooperative Study Group on Anti-hypertensive Agents, led by Dr. Edward Freis; initial results were published in 1967 (Veterans Administration Cooperative Study Group, 1967). In this report 143 male hypertensive patients whose unmedicated diastolic BP had consistently been between 115 and 129 mm Hg were randomized to either a drug regimen comprised of reserpine, hydrochlorothiazide and hydralazine, or matched placebo. Care had been taken before the study began to eliminate patients with more serious hypertension and severe-end organ damage, those who were apparently noncompliant during a 2-month placebo phase prior to beginning the study, and those of "dubious reliability." With this screening, only 12 patients dropped out over the 3 years of the study. Average age of the sample was 50.7 years; it was 53% black.

It had been planned to follow patients for 5 years after they began therapy. The study was stopped after 3 years: Active drug therapy had averaged 21 months while placebo therapy averaged only 16 months. The BP changes were dramatic: The treated group's SBP dropped an average of 43 mm Hg while DBP decreased 30 mm Hg. The average BPs of the placebo group did not change.

Four patients in the placebo group died versus none on active therapy. Ten additional placebo-treated patients had such serious illnesses that they were removed from the study, as were 7 others whose BP continued to increase. Only one drug-treated patient was removed from the study, the cause was progression of BP. This difference in morbidity and mortality was significant at $p < .001$. The results were so dramatic in such a relatively short period (average participation of less than 2 years) that the trial was halted. It was seen as unethical to continue patients on the placebo.

It had thus been shown clearly that reducing the BP of patients with severe hypertension made striking differences in morbidity and mortality. In fact, the risk can be established for this group as 0.29 morbid events/man-year. This means that in 10 men with DBPs in this range who are untreated for 1 year, one could expect 3 of the 10 to have a serious hypertension-related illness.

1970 VA Cooperative Study

The other arm of the VA Cooperative Study (VA Cooperative Study Group, 1970) contained 380 males whose entry DBPs ranged from 90 to 114 mm Hg. They received the same drug regimen (hydrochlorothiazide, reserpine, and hydralazine). This group was about the same age (51.2 years), but only 41.3% black. BPs on entry averaged 164/104. Patients were followed on average for 3.25 years.

Therapy was again effective on BP: the treated group's BPs fell by 27.2 mm SBP and 17.4 mm DBP, compared with an increase of 4.2/1.2 mm for the placebo controls. Dropouts were evenly distributed and amounted to 15%.

There were 19 deaths (9.8%) in the placebo group, compared with 8 (4.3%) of those in active therapy; 5 of the 19 were due to stroke, while 14 were due to coronary heart disease. In the treated group all 8 deaths were due to coronary heart disease. Total morbid events, such as congestive heart failure, stroke, or progression of elevated BP, were 76 for the placebo patients versus 22 for the treated patients, a highly significant difference. Based on a life-table analysis, projected to 5 years, the placebo group could have expected a morbid event rate of 55%, versus only 18% for treated patients, a difference significant at $p < .001$.

Subsample analyses showed a greater advantage for treatment over placebo for patients whose entering DBP was 105 to 114 than for those with DBPs of 90 to 104. In fact, for these patients with mild hypertension, the difference in rate of morbid events for treated versus placebo (16.3% versus 25.0%, respectively) was not significant.

This study thus showed that there was demonstrable advantage for treatment of moderate hypertension (DBP of 105–114 mm Hg) and that the advantage was primarily in the prevention of stroke and congestive heart failure rather than coronary artery disease.

Hypertension Detection and Follow-up Program

The next major study in this area was the Hypertension Detection and Follow-up Program (HDFP) (HDFP Cooperative Group, 1976; 1979a, 1979b; 1982a, 1982b). It targeted patients from the community with mild hypertension (90–104 mm Hg). In addition to the targeted population, several other features of HDFP were markedly different from the VA Cooperative Study: (1) The control group, rather than receiving a placebo, were referred to their usual source of care in the community (Referred Care [RC]), while the experimental group received drugs according to a series of steps (Stepped Care [SC]) of increasing number and types of drugs in order to bring DBP below 90 mm Hg; (2) the sample sizes were increased by a factor of 20, such that 7825 patients with mild hypertension were randomized to SC or RC.

At a 5-year follow-up, 63.8% of the Stepped Care patients had DBPs in the normotensive range versus 43.0% of those in RC. Average DBPs for the two groups at 5 years were 83.4 mm for SC versus 87.8 mm for RC. Much of the difference in mortality was in stroke and CHD (HDFP Cooperative Group, 1979a, 1979b). The overall 5-year death rates (mortality) for the experimental group (SC) was 5.9/100 versus 7.4/100 for those in RC, a significant advantage for SC of 20.3% ($p < .01$).

It thus took much larger samples to show a statistically significant advantage for SC over RC for mortality rates in mild hypertension than with patients with more severe disease.

Further analyses by substrata showed trends for Stepped Care to have an advantage over RC for those with entry DBPs of 90–94 mm, (n = 2941, p = .08) and of 95–100 (n = 2731, 23.1%, p = .10) (HDFP Cooperative Group, 1982b). Taken as a whole, these results seemed to indicate that there is an advantage in treating even mild hypertension. However, Freis (1982) called that conclusion into question, especially the extrapolation that one should perhaps treat patients with high normal (85–89 mm Hg) DBPs since treatment "condemned the patient to a life time of drug therapy" with its possible risks and costs in absence of clearly established benefits.

Australian National Blood Pressure Study

Contemporaneous with HDFP in the USA another large-scale trial was being conducted in Australia (Management Committee, Australian National Blood Pressure Study, 1980); 3427 men and women with mild hypertension were randomized to active antihypertensive therapy or placebo and followed for 4 years. Approximately one third dropped out, leaving 2218 followed on therapy for 4 years. (Eligibility for this study, and thus the definition of mild hypertension, was DBPs between 95 and 109 mm Hg.)

The treated patients (including drop-outs) had a lower (p < .05) overall death rate (1.7/1000 person years) than did the placebo patients including drop-outs (3.7/1000). There were also significantly (p < .025) reduced morbidity from all cardiovascular disease 15.5/1000 person years (for treated) versus 20.8/1000 for placebo patients.

Thus, these results seem to replicate the main findings of HDFP in a somewhat different population (HDFP had more patients with complications such as diabetes entering the trial) and with a different design (placebo-controlled rather than RC): Treatment of mild hypertension does reduce morbidity and mortality.

Multiple-Risk-Factor Intervention Trial (MRFIT)

Although the central theme of the previous research seemed fairly straight forward, reduction of elevated BP reduces morbidity and mortality, even in mild hypertension, the majority of the reductions were in stroke and other cardiovascular disease rather than in coronary heart disease (CHD). Contemporaneous with the HDFP, the National Heart, Lung and Blood Institute (NHLBI) also launched a major effort to see if the morbidity and mortality associated with CHD could be prevented by intervening in known risk factors for CHD. The risk factors to the targeted were identified in large part from the findings of the Framingham studies and included elevated DBP, cigarette smoking, and elevated serum cholesterol.

Thus, the MRFIT was launched with 12,866 men shown to be at high risk for CHD based on the above three risk factors. Half were randomized to a Special Intervention (SI) program designed to reduce the levels in the three risk factors, while the others were referred to their own physician for the Usual Level of Care (UC) while being reexamined yearly. All patients were followed for at least 6 years with an average of 7 years (MRFIT Research Group, 1982).

Treatment of hypertension was through a stepped-care drug regimen similar to that used in HDFP. Diastolic BP was reduced from an average screening level of 99 mm Hg (and an average baseline level of 91 mm Hg) to 80.5 mm Hg by year 6. By year 4 (Cohen, Grimm & Smith, 1981) 83.5% of the hypertensives assigned to the SI condition had DBPs below 90 mm Hg.

The Special Intervention group showed significantly greater ($p < .01$) reductions on all three risk factors than did the UC group at each yearly check-up. Despite the success of the interventions *there were no differences* in overall mortality rate or in mortality due to CHD between the SI and UC groups (MRFIT Research Group, 1982).

Interestingly, there were no significant advantages for SI over UC in terms of CHD to deaths for any DBP level (90–94, 95–99, 100+), despite overall greater reductions in DBP levels in the Special Intervention group. One anomalous, and somewhat alarming, finding was the *higher* CHD death rate for patients in the SI condition among the subset of hypertensives who entered the trial with various ECG abnormalities (19% of total sample): 29.2/1000 over 6 years for SI versus 17.7/1000 for UC (MRFIT Research Group, 1982).

It thus appears that for a sizeable proportion of male hypertensives, aggressive drug treatment of BP may not be in their best interest. The drug regimen may interact with existing ECG abnormalities. In any event, this finding has led to some caution in blanket attempts to lower BP with drugs, especially in those with very mild hypertension. It probably served as part of the impetus for the point made in the next section.

Assistant Secretary for Health's Advisory (1983)

In 1983 Brandt, the Assistant Secretary for Health (of Department of Health and Human Services), issued an advisory based upon the above findings that is relevant to the purpose of this book:

> I would like to reinforce that mild hypertension should not be ignored. I believe the following . . . constitute prudent practice.
>
> Initiate treatment of mild high blood pressure, particularly in the range of 90–94 mm Hg diastolic pressure, *with nonpharmacologic measures* [italics added] as long as this treatment is effective in maintaining normal blood pressure . . . .
>
> In general, it is prudent medical therapy to *use the lowest dosage of any drug* [italics added] effective in maintaining control . . . . (p. 25)

SUMMARY

As an answer to the rhetorical question—"why we should treat hypertension"—which began this section, we can say that it has been clearly established for 15 years that antihypertensive drug therapy reduces morbidity and mortality in those with moderate or severe hypertension. For those with mild hypertension, this same conclusion has been warranted since 1980 (however, the strength of the advantage is more modest). It appears that immediate aggressive pharmacotherapy for everyone with mild hypertension is not necessarily the best choice and that a reasonable trial of nonpharmacological therapy, the topic of this book, is warranted.

Chapter 2

Physiology of Blood Pressure

Thus far, we have described why elevated blood pressure is so dangerous, and who tends to develop the disorder of hypertension. In this chapter we will provide a little more detail regarding what high blood pressure is, including the physiological mechanisms for the control of blood pressure. We should first make it clear, however, that we do not know precisely why people develop hypertension—though we do understand that it occurs more frequently in blacks, as well as in those who are more overweight/overfat, sedentary, and who have a higher intake of salt in their diet. Subsequent chapters will address how we can lower high blood pressure by attacking these risk factors with behavioral interventions; in this chapter we hope to provide the clinician with a basic knowledge of how blood pressure works and what may go wrong.

The Physiology of Blood Pressure

Blood pressure, simply, is the pressure generated within the cardiovascular system—the heart, arteries, veins and capillaries—during the beating and resting phases of the heart. For our purposes, a good analogy is the water pump, although the cardiovascular system is indeed much more complex than that. Generally, the heart pumps the available blood into the arteries—the pipes of our hydraulic system model. We measure this pressure, as will be detailed in the next chapter, by occluding or blocking this blood flow at a convenient place (the upper arm usually) and measuring the pressure (a) at which the heart is able to pump the blood past the temporary barrier (blood pressure cuff) (systolic blood pressure, SBP), and (b) at the resting steady state, between beats of the heart (diastolic blood pressure, DBP; i.e., the pressure exerted on the arm by the cuff and the blood pressure are the same).

The simplest and probably the most widely acknowledged explanation of blood pressure regulation (especially among psychologists, e.g., Surwit, Williams, & Shapiro, 1982) reveals two essentially independent components that interact to produce ultimate blood pressure. This mechanical model explains control of the blood pressure level both at rest (DBP) and during the contraction of the heart muscle (SBP) through a linear interaction between the variables that make up these two basic components. This relationship can be stated in its simplest form as follows: AP = CO × TPR where AP is arterial pressure, CO is cardiac output (determined by the fluid volume and the pumping action of the heart), and TPR is total peripheral resistance (made up of vascular factors causing relative dilation or constriction of the blood vessels). A closer look at the two components of arterial pressure is important both to an appreciation of the complexity of even this simplified formula and to a general understanding of the relationship of diet, stress, and physical exercise to the normal functioning of human blood pressure.

Cardiac output. A number of factors can alter overall cardiac output. Broadly, anything that changes the volume of blood and fluid, or the rate at which it is transported in the circulatory system, should change blood pressure. Thus, increases in the circulatory fluid volume or in the viscosity of the blood should, all other things remaining equal, result in increased blood pressure. Likewise, anything that alters the rate at which the heart pumps the total volume of blood and fluid from the heart into the arteries will proportionately change pressure. For example, psychological or physical stress are both likely to increase both heart rate and stroke volume (the amount of blood expelled from the main pumping station, the left ventricle, of the heart on a beat; this volume measure is determined by the force exerted upon each contraction of the heart muscle) through sympathetic neurohormone activity, and thereby lead to an increase in blood pressure (Surwit et al., 1982).

Total peripheral resistance. The other part of the equation looks at the space through which the volume of fluid is being pushed. Logically, anything that serves to constrict or narrow the vascular pathways should also serve to increase blood pressure. For example, psychological stress can cause an increase in sympathetic activity, which, in turn, may produce a pressor response—an abrupt increase in peripheral resistance through constriction of the blood vessels. In part, this pressor reaction, producing an almost immediate spike in blood pressure, is an exceedingly important adaptive response to threat, injury, or other profound anticipated physical effort (e.g., hunting, mating). For example, threat of injury or actual injury (e.g., puncture) might result in much more severe blood loss or death in the absence of vasoconstriction, which shunts the blood supply away from the periphery to the more central vital organs. If this response becomes chronic, hypertension might theoretically follow.

Another relatively common cause of increased total peripheral resistance relates to the chronic rather than acute narrowing of the blood vessels: Depositing of fat on the interior lining of the blood vessel walls. This coronary and peripheral vascular occlusive process can be attributed mainly to diets high in cholesterol and saturated fat, and to some extent stress (e.g., Type A Behavior Pattern) which may ultimately result in elevated blood pressure due to chronic increases in TPR. In addition, smoking (principally carbon monoxide in the inhaled smoke) is associated with accelerations in this clogging of the blood vessels through enhancing the attachment of fat deposits to the vessel walls.

THE REST OF THE STORY

A Systems Theory of Blood Pressure Control

Unfortunately, blood pressure does not appear to operate so simply. Although it is generally accurate and helpful to our initial under-standing, the major difficulty with the linear mechanical model (AP = CO × TPR) is that its component parts are not, in fact, independent (Guyton, 1980). Further, more recent and comprehensive data suggest a much more important role for the kidney, and for the process of *autoregulation* than had previously been suspected, and a less important role for stress/high-blood-pressure theories, so popular in the psychological and early behavioral medicine literature, in the long-term control of blood pressure (Guyton, 1980).

Dynamic systems theories of blood pressure regulation, such as presented by Guyton (1980), go an important step beyond the linear mechanics shown in the previous section and acknowledge the fact that CO and TPR are intimately connected and interdependent (Hollandsworth, 1986). For example, because the heart is much like a sump pump that pumps out all the blood that is fed into it, increasing TPR will feed less fluid back to the heart, thereby reducing CO (Hollandsworth, 1986). This leads to a much more complex formulation to predict blood pressure.

Buffering mechanisms. We know that hypertension is rarely due to increases in sympathetic activity (e.g., stress) alone (Guyton, 1980). In our blood pressure regulatory system, there are numerous checks and balances designed to attenuate and ultimately neutralize the effect of heightened arousal (e.g., high heart rate). In the normal individual, there are several buffering mechanisms that "kick in" when blood pressure is detected that is too high or low. The baroreceptor buffering mechanism, for instance, detects pressure changes through the stretching of the blood vessels. In the event there is too much stretch (BP too high) or too little (BP too low), the baroreceptors communicate more or less directly with the sympathetic activation system and the blood vessels (vagal impulses) to countermand the direction of the blood pressure. That is, if pressure is getting too high, the vessels are dilated and the sympathetic stimulation to the heart is decreased to lower pressure.

Another buffering mechanism that is of utmost importance to the regulation of blood pressure is the hormonal buffering mechanism of the renin-angiotensin system. It is maximally effective in the blood pressure ranges between 50 and 90 mm Hg and is primarily responsible for *increasing* blood pressure that has fallen too much, too quickly (i.e., to prevent death from shock or blood loss). When low pressures are detected, renin is liberated, which in turn liberates angiotensin, which causes significant vasoconstriction. Importantly, this renin-angiotensin-vasoconstriction response chain may also be invoked through sympathetic overarousal.

Unfortunately, in hypertensives these protective buffering mechanisms may adapt to the new, higher blood pressure levels, and cease to function, or they may reset to higher levels, thereby maintaining too high a pressure in the system. More on this process later.

The role of the kidneys. The kidneys have two main functions in life: (1) to eliminate waste products from the blood and (2) to regulate blood pressure. Most of the other mechanisms for blood pressure control (especially the cardiosympathetic) discussed previously have been shown to be relatively short-acting regulators of blood pressure, acting nearly instantaneously up to about 72 hours. The kidneys, on the other hand, are designed in part to regulate blood pressure over the long run through a process of fluid/sodium/electrolyte retention and expulsion. Hence, if blood pressure is too high, natural mechanisms within the blood vessels of the kidneys activate a process that purges increasing amounts of fluid and electrolytes (such as the fluid-holding sodium) until the blood pressure is normalized.

This renal function curve (Guyton, 1980) is set at normal limits and will cause corrective action if blood pressure ventures above or below these preset normal limits. No matter how high the blood pressure goes, in the normal individual the kidneys are capable of (and ultimately responsible for) normalizing the pressure through fluid adjustments (i.e., they control the water pressure release valve!). In some cases, however, this renal function curve is abnormally reset higher and higher in response to changes in the system (such as diet, weight and physical activity) that drive up blood pressure, and chronic hypertension can result. For example, we know that increased amounts of sodium in the diet can result in increased blood pressure through affecting renal function and consequent fluid retention.

It is important to note that the renal/blood-pressure-control system can also be affected by neural/sympathetic activation. An excellent example of how sympathetic activation can act through the renal pathway to alter blood pressure is provided by Light, Koepke, Obrist, and Willis (1983). They found that in individuals who had been preloaded with fluid, psychological stress resulted in a hypertensive effect of increasing fluid retention (kidney output restricted). Interestingly, physical stress (treadmill work) had the opposite effect; that is, lowering blood pressure due to enhancing the kidney functions of fluid and electrolyte purging.

Metabolic processes. A final but very important component in the blood pressure system we have been discussing incorporates the body's metabolic regulation system. This may be loosely divided into the carbohydrate and lipid (breakdown) metabolic system and the tissue (sustenance) autoregulation system. Recent research has indicated the importance of *insulin, carbohydrate and lipid metabolism* to blood pressure, especially in the overweight (Krotkiewski et al., 1979; Sims, 1982). In addition, it appears that overweight hypertensives are especially likely to have hyperinsulinemia and hyperlipidemia, as well as relatively poor glucose tolerance, and that these metabolic abnormalities may well be associated with the development of the hypertension. At the very least, the high blood pressure may be maintained by these metabolic dys-functions. Similarly, the ingestion of even moderate amounts of alcohol has also been associated with elevated pressures in some individuals (Joint National Committee on Detection, Evaluation and Treatment of High Blood Pressure, 1986), possibly due to its relationship with overweight, but more likely resulting from further disturbance in the metabolic-breakdown process. Finally, hyperinsulinemia has been shown to negatively affect renal function, and sodium reabsorption and retention (Simms, 1982), thereby adding to the already complex metabolic/blood-pressure-regulatory disturbance.

Another important but little-understood process in the blood pressure regulation system has been termed *autoregulation* (Guyton, 1980). Essentially, *metabolic autoregulation* is the process by which tissue systematically adjusts the perfusion of its needed nutrients and oxygen through vasoconstriction/vasodilation of the arterioles—the most important determinant of TPR (Guyton, 1980). As noted by Hollandsworth (1986), the most important point to remember is that this process is not mediated neurally, but rather by the metabolic requirements of the tissue (probably oxygen or blood pH).

These recent findings regarding the importance of renal function and autoregulation for blood pressure control tend to shift our attention away from the somewhat disappointing, if not inadequate, autonomic nervous system explanations, to a more balanced picture. If hypertension is to be *comprehensively* treated, it would make sense then to incorporate each of these component systems into our treatment system in order to ensure long-term as well as the short-term control of blood pressure.

Physiology of Hypertension: An Interaction of Systems

Because the circulatory system, including the heart and all the blood vessels, is essentially a closed system, any changes in the system components (such as heart rate or kidney output) have the potential to alter blood pressure. In the event that a correcting change is not elicited in a countercontrolling component of the system (e.g., vasodilation following heart rate increase) to recalibrate blood pressure to normal, high blood pressure can result.

It should be stated at this point that the blood-pressure-normalizing components built into the system are designed to be powerful and effective, and includes numerous back-up systems (remember that blood pressure must be maintained within certain limits to ensure survival). Basically there are four general systems we have discussed that work toward this end—the cardiosympathetic system, the renal function/fluid regulation system, the metabolic processing and regulation systems, and the interactive buffering systems. Individually they exert powerful control in regulating blood pressure; together their influence would seem insurmountable, no matter what the internal or external conditions. Unfortunately, sometimes extraordinary conditions come in to play that over the long run undermine these potent blood pressure control systems, and hypertension results.

Although the interactions of these blood pressure regulation systems can be quite complex, generally when one component functions abnormally (or is subjected to abnormal or significant pressure from other external or internal sources) it often requires other balancing systems to malfunction before hypertension results. Yet, as we know, this scenario too frequently occurs. Importantly, this disregulation of blood pressure can be related to the interplay of physiological control mechanisms noted previously, of undampened cardiosympathetic overarousal, renal dysfunction, maladaptive (in terms of blood pressure) metabolic processing and autoregulation, and inadequate mechanical, neural, and hormonal buffering.

From systems to persons. Although we have yet to identify a gene that carries the disease of hypertension, we do know that it tends to run in families (a weak predictor, however), certain racial groups (blacks), and appears in certain environments more frequently (high stress/industrialized). More often, however, it is associated with specific acquired personal characteristics (overweight) and behaviors (diet, poor stress/coping, physical inactivity)—which will be discussed in the following chapters. When these variables interact, as they often do, in susceptible individuals the blood pressure regulation mechanisms can be further defeated—not just over the short run (e.g., stress-induced accute tachycardia and blood pressure elevation), but over the long run as well—to produce, or increasingly maintain, chronic essential hypertension.

As the following chapters will illustrate, specific psychological and behavioral interventions that target these modifiable characteristics and behavior patterns may serve to countermand, if not correct, the disregulated blood pressure system. As an illustration of this point, consider the following: Exercise can result not only in a chronic lowering of heart rate, but more importantly in an adaptive increase in kidney function and output, and enhancement of autoregulatory perfusion (to meet the increased metabolic demands of the enlarging vascularization of lean tissue mass), as well as improvements in hyperinsulinemia, hyperlipidemia and glucose tolerance. On top of all this, and partly as a general consequence, a chronic dilation of the blood vessels may also be experienced.

These system changes as a result of exercise may together serve to ultimately lower resting (and possibly active) blood pressure levels through normalizing the system components that initially failed in response to the hypertensive challenge from internal and external factors. Similarly profound effects of dietary and stress-management therapy are also possible, especially given the intimate interdependence of the system components that are affected by these nondrug therapies. A case in point is the striking finding of Light et al. (1983) indicating the sensitive interplay between the sympathetic activation and renal control systems (among others), and the consequent importance of individual volitional, behavioral components such as stress coping, diet, and physical activity in the checks and balances of the overall blood pressure regulatory system.

As will be seen in subsequent chapters, exercise, stress management, and dietary interventions may work through a variety of system pathways and components to alter the blood pressure disregulation, perhaps through rebalancing the distorted system. We believe the remainder of the book will provide some useful strategies regarding assessing and modifying the critical characteristics and behavior patterns of stress responding, diet, and physical inactivity, which can produce and/or help maintain hypertension in susceptible individuals.

Chapter 3

Assessment Procedures: History Taking, Blood Pressure Measurement and Psychological Testing

TAKING A COMPREHENSIVE HISTORY

In this chapter we describe basic initial assessment procedures that should probably be conducted on all patients: (a) a comprehensive history; (b) careful measurement of blood pressure; and (c) psychological testing. (We also admit that there may not be universal agreement on the need for the last procedure but have included it nonetheless.)

In concert with standard medical and psychological practice, we believe the first step in the nonpharmacological treatment of the hypertensive patient should be the taking of a good history. In our experience, almost all hypertensives present for nonpharmacological treatment knowing their diagnosis as a result of previous medical examination. Thus, diagnosis and differential diagnosis are not the primary goals in taking a history. Instead, the therapist is seeking to gather information for several other purposes: (a) as a way of establishing a relationship with the patient; (b) to gather information that may have some value in predicting treatment outcome; (c) to gather information possibly relevant to the particular treatment strategy to be used; (d) to have an adequate understanding of the patient and the patient's hypertension; (e) to screen for other psychological problems which may need attention in the course of treating the whole patient.

19

The history form described below is designed to meet all of these purposes. In addition, there are sections designed to gather information specific to one of the three primary intervention modalities: stress management, dietary changes, or exercise.

The Importance of Close Medical Collaboration

We cannot stress too strongly the need for close medical collaboration in this work. (We are assuming that most users of this *Guidebook* are not physicians.) Unless you happen to be engaged in the unlikely task of screening a large number of individuals for elevated BP in a setting such as the work site, the vast majority of your patients will come to you with the diagnosis of hypertension having previously been made by a medical facility or physician. Many will come on direct referral by their physician to you for nonpharmacological treatment.

In our opinion, the nonphysician practitioner should not begin treatment of the hypertensive patient until that patient has had a thorough physical examination and the diagnosis of essential hypertension is confirmed. There are many potential causes of elevated BP such as pheochromocytoma and renal disease that need to be diagnosed and handled by the physician.

An overriding rule of thumb: do not attempt to diagnose and treat outside of your area of expertise!

Antihypertensive medications. Patients will obviously present to you in one of three states: (a) with elevated BP but not on antihypertensive medication; (b) on antihypertensive medication with BP under control; or (c) on antihypertensive medication but with BP still elevated. The management of the antihypertensive drugs in these three cases is somewhat different; all cases require close cooperation with the prescribing or referring physician.

Elevated BP, no meds. The majority of patients in this category will have only mild hypertension (defined as DBP between 90 and 104 mm Hg). As noted in Chapter 1, there is some risk associated with having one's BP in this range and not receiving therapy to reduce it. However, that risk is small and probably acceptable for a trial of up to 3 months of nondrug therapy, especially if the patient has no other major risk factors for coronary heart disease. (If the DBP is in the range of 90–95 and there are no other major risk factors, one could probably extend the nondrug time to 6 months. Again be guided in part by close collaboration with the referring physician.)

If BP has not been reduced within 3 to 6 months, or if DBP rises to consistently above 104 mm Hg, the patient should probably be considered a failure and should be referred back to the physician for drug therapy.

Elevated BP, on meds. Patients in this category and in the next one both present a potentially tricky liaison problem in that one goal of therapy is the reduction of antihypertensive medication, as well as the reduction of BP. Close monitoring of BP is strongly advised. As therapy succeeds and BP begins to decrease to within the normotensive range, it would be good if the patient could gradually reduce the antihypertensive medications. Reduction of antihypertensive medication is a potentially strong and powerful reinforcer for the patient! Supervision of this drug reduction should be in the hands of the physician, *not the patient* and *not the nonmedical therapist*.

If possible, a schedule of appointments for BP checks and medication changes should be arranged with the prescribing physician (perhaps monthly) so that close titration of the drug dosage and good overall liaison are maintained. If this close liaison is not possible (e.g., the physician does not want to see the patient until you are through), then remind the patient to return to the physician at the end of treatment.

Meds; no elevation in BP. This patient is probably coming with the goal of reducing or eliminating antihypertensive medication. In addition to the liaison issues described above, a potential problem in this case is that BP becomes so low that the patient begins to have symptoms because of the low BP (hypotension). Such symptoms could be fatigue and dizziness, especially dizziness when standing up suddenly. One should probably strive harder for close liaison in this case than in the one above.

You should probably check back with the physician yourself at the end of treatment to be sure the patient has made contact. This crosschecking can prevent having a patient "slip through the cracks." It might also be wise to send the physician a letter summarizing treatment and BPs.

Hypertension History Forms

In this section we present forms for taking an initial history from the hypertensive patient. Table 3–1 presents a basic demographic data sheet we have found useful. In Table 3–2 is the basic history form used in the Stress Disorders Clinic at SUNY-Albany, modified to include basic informational items used at the Jackson VAMC. Tables 3–3 through 3–5 are specific addenda from the Jackson VAMC designed to gather

Table 3-1. Basic Demographic Data Sheet

Date _____

1. Name _____
2. Current address _____
   _____
3. Telephone number(s): Home _____
   Work _____ Other _____
4. Age _____ Birth date _____
5. Marital status _____
6. Sex _____
7. Occupation (current) _____
   (previous) _____
8. Years of education _____
9. Approximate annual income _____
10. Current living arrangements (persons in household and their relationship to patient)
    _____

11. Name and address of someone who will always know how to contact patient
    _____

12. Referral source (From whom or what did you hear about the project?)
    _____

13. Personal physician (name and address) _____
    _____

14. Brief history of hypertension:
    a. How long: _____
    b. Medication taken: (past)   _____
    c.   (present) _____
    d. Any related medical problems _____
    _____

    e. Any prescription medications other than antihypertension medication:
    _____

15. Current blood pressure as measured in office _____/_____ _____
                                                                        Date
                                                 _____/_____ _____
                                                                        Date

information that would be useful for exercise programs (3–3), dietary interventions (3–4), as well as a few questions on smoking (3–5).

Table 3–2 is designed to elicit the history of the patient's hypertension and any drug therapy received for it. It next seeks to gather data in the form of a behavioral analysis to see if the patient is aware of fluctuations in BP and of environmental reactions to this problem. We also try to gather a fairly detailed description of current social situations and potential psychological problems. It concludes with a brief mental-status examination. Most of the items in this table are set up for easy computing-coding, as is obvious from the material on the right-hand side of the page.

The exercise-related questions in Table 3–3 are designed to gain a history of previous attempts at a regular aerobic exercise program and to

Table 3-2. Hypertension Interview

Code key: 1 = Yes; 0 = No; 8 = No knowledge; 9 = N/A, unless otherwise specified.

1. When were you first diagnosed as having high blood pressure? (age and number of years ago)	Age No. of yrs. ago No	____ ____ ____
2. Was the onset, as far as you can tell, associated with any particular stressful event (physical or psychological) in your life? Describe _____	Physical illness Psychosocial event Pregnancy Other	____ ____ ____ ____
3. a. Have you been under medical care for hypertension continuously since that time?	a.	____
b. What sorts of medications have you received in the past to treat your hypertension?	b. Diuretics Symp. Blockers Vasodilators Others	____ ____ ____ ____
c. What medications are you currently taking for hypertension? ·	c. Diuretic, etc.	____
d. Have you ever, on your own initiative, or by doctor's directions, discontinued taking hypertension medications for any period of time?	d.	
e. Why?	e. Expense Side effects Ineffective Forgot Other	____ ____ ____ ____ ____
4. What is the highest your blood pressure has ever been?	Systolic Diastolic	__ __ __ __ __ __
5. Is it higher in the doctor's office than at home?	0 = No; 2 = Yes; 1 = Sometimes	____
a. Are you aware of events in your environment that cause your blood pressure to fluctuate? (Short term = same day)	Short-term Long-term	____ ____
b. What events?	a. Physical illness Physical injury Psychosocial event Menstrual cycle Pregnancy Job stress Other	____ ____ ____ ____ ____ ____ ____
6. Are there any sensations you become aware of when your blood pressure is higher than usual?	0 = No; 1 = Sometimes; 2 = Yes, definitely	____
a. How?	Muscle tension Nervousness Pounding heart Headache Dizziness Nosebleeds Excessive perspiration Other	____ ____ ____ ____ ____ ____ ____ ____

Table 3-2. *Continued*

b. Are there any sensations you become
   aware of when your blood pressure is   0 = No; 1 = Maybe;
   lower than usual?   2 = Yes, definitely   ____
c. How?   Dizziness/lightheadedness   ____
                                               Weakness   ____
                                               Sense of well-being   ____
                                               Other   ____

7. Once you have taken your blood pressure   0 = Nothing   ____
   and discovered it is higher than usual, what 1 = Internal (what did I do?);
   are your reactions, thoughts, feelings?   2 = External (why me?);
                                               3 = Other

Consequences of Hypertension

8. When you realize your blood pressure is   0 = Nothing; 1 = Something   ____
   higher than usual, do you do anything?
   a. If so, what?   Call doctor   ____
                                               Try to relax, (avoid activities) ____
                                               Alter meds on your own   ____
                                               Other   ____

9. How often do you get your blood pressure checked? _____
   Where? _____
10. Do you have any objections to taking medication? Yes _____ No _____
    If yes, what? _____
    _____

11. Do you have trouble swallowing the pills? Yes ____ No ____ Sometimes ____
12. Where do you get your medication/refills? _____
13. How do you order refills? _____
14. How many times per day do you *actually* take your medication? _____
15. How do you remember to take it? _____
16. How often do you actually forget to take it? _____
17. When was the last time you forgot to take your medication? _____
18. Have situations arisen when you have not been able to take your medication?
    (such as being away from home, running out of medication, etc.)?
    Yes _____ No _____
19. What is the longest period of time you have forgotten or not taken your medication?
    _____
20. How long have you been taking medicine for your high blood pressure? _____
21. How does the medication make you feel? Any side effects? Yes _____ No _____
    What type of side effects? _____
22. Can you afford to buy your medication? Yes _____ No_____
23. What do your family/friends say about your taking medicine? _____
    _____

24. Does your hypertension interfere with your   0 = No; 1 = Somewhat;
    daily life?   2 = Yes, definitely
    a. How?   Miss school or work   ____
                                                 Slow down or become less
                                                    efficient   ____
                                                 Forgo recreational activities ____
                                                 Other   ____
25. Do you tell significant others when your
    blood pressure is unusually high?
    a. Can they tell without your mentioning it?   ____

Table 3-2. *Continued*

26. Do they react to this knowledge? _____
    How?   Express concern _____
                                    Offer help _____
                                    Nag _____
                                    Other _____
27. Other than taking medication do you do
    anything to prevent increases in your blood
    pressure?
    a. What?   Try to relax _____
                                    Watch diet _____
                                    Avoid strenuous activity _____
                                    Other _____
28. As you know, hypertension sometimes runs   (Use this code for all parts
    in families. Are you aware of blood pressure   of this question)
    problems, heart disease or heart attack,
    stroke, kidney disease?   0 = No _____
                                    1 = Essential hypertension _____
                                    2 = Kidney _____
                                    3 = Stroke _____
                                    4 = Heart attack _____
                                    5 = Other _____
    a. In mother _____
    b. Father _____
    c. Grandparents _____
    d. Siblings _____
    e. Children _____
    f. Blood relatives _____
29. Now I need some information on your current
    life situation.   Married _____
    a. If married, how would you describe your _____
       marriage?   0 = Excellent
                                    1 = Good
                                    2 = Average/normal
                                    3 = Poor/problems
                                    9 = N/A
    b. Are you getting along well?
    c. Are there any problems? If yes, ask for   Communication _____
       details.   Financial _____
                                    Affairs _____
                                    Situational factors _____
                                    Illness _____
                                    Other _____
                                    N/A = 9 _____
    d. How is your sexual relationship?
                                    0 = Excellent
                                    1 = Good
                                    2 = Normal/average
                                    3 = Poor/problems
                                    9 = N/A
    e. Are there any problems?   0 = No; 1 = Yes; 9 = N/A _____
                                    Sexual dysfunction _____
                                    Physical illness/injury _____
                                    Lack of interest of one
                                       partner _____
                                    Other _____

Table 3-2. *Continued*

f. Do you have any problems with your
in-laws?   ____

g. Do you have any problems with parents?   ____

h. (If patient has children, regardless of
marital status)
Are there any problems with your
children?   ____

30. If not married, are you currently involved in
some sort of relationship?   ____

a. Are you getting along well?   ____

b. Are there any problems?   ____
(If yes, ask for details.)   Communication   ____
                                           Financial   ____
                                           Affairs   ____
                                           Illness   ____

c. Is there a sexual aspect to your   Sexual dysfunction   ____
relationship? (If yes, are there any   Physical illness/injury   ____
problems here?)   Lack of interest of one
                                              partner   ____
                                           Other   ____

d. Do you have any problems with your
parents?   ____

31. Do you have some close friends?   ____
How many really close friends?   ____
Have there been any difficulties in   ____
friendships?   ____

32. (If patient works or attends school)
How are you getting along with your job   0 = Excellent
(schoolwork)?   1 = Good
                                           2 = Average/normal
                                           3 = Poor/problems
                                           9 = N/A (retired)

a. Are there any problems?   ____
Especially with supervisors (or teachers)?   ____
If yes, how are you handling these   Ignoring/avoiding   ____
problems?   Arguing   ____
                                           Rational discussion   ____

b. Do you feel under a lot of pressure in your   ____
job (or schoolwork)?   0 = No
                                           1 = Yes
                                           2 = Sometimes
                                           3 = N/A

c. Does this seem related to high blood   ____
pressure? (How?)   0 = No
                                           1 = Yes
                                           2 = Sometimes
                                           3 = N/A

33. These next few questions may seem   0 = Correct
somewhat strange, but bear with me.   1 = Incorrect
What is today's date? The day of the week?
Do you remember my name?   ____
I am going to say some numbers; listen   ____
carefully, then repeat them back to me (give
digits approximately one per second, do not
repeat)

Table 3-2. *Continued*

(i) 5–8–2 (ii) 6–9–4 (iii) 6–4–3–9	0 = Only 3 digits correct	_____
(iv) 7–2–8–6 (v) 4–2–7–3–1	1 = 3 & 4 digits correct	
(vi) 7–5–8–3–6	2 = All correct	
Who is the President of the U.S.?	0 = Correct	_____
Who is the Governor of New York	1 = Incorrect	_____
Have you ever had any strange experiences?		_____
Have you ever heard things other people could not hear or heard things when no one was there?		_____
Have you ever seen things that other people could not see?		_____
Do you believe you have special powers?		_____
Have you ever felt or thought people were out to get you?		_____
Have you ever been depressed?		_____
If yes, are you depressed now?		_____
If yes, check further.	Sleep disturbance	_____
	Loss of appetite/weight	_____
	Loss of concentration	_____
	Anhedonia	_____
	Loss of interest in sex	_____
	Low energy	_____
	Suicidal ideation	_____
	Suicidal attempts made	_____
34. Have you ever been really "speeded up," had a great deal of energy, didn't need much sleep?		_____
Have you ever had a problem with alcohol or with other drugs?		_____
35. Have you ever received any psychiatric or psychological treatment for mental or emotional problems?		_____
If yes, obtain brief details including current status of treatment.	*Currently in treatment* 0 = No, 1 = Yes, 9 = N/A	_____
	Treatment terminated 0 = No, 1 = Yes, 9 = N/A	_____
	Treatment helpful 0 = No, 1 = Yes, 9 = N/A	_____
	Treatment not helpful 0 = No, 1 = Yes, 9 = N/A	_____
36. Have you ever had major illnesses or operations:	0 = No, 1 = Yes	_____
Obtain details	*Major operations* 0 = No, 1 = Yes, 9 = N/A	_____
	Major illnesses 0 = No, 1 = Yes, 9 = N/A	_____
	Chronic illness 0 = No, 1 = Yes, 9 = N/A	_____
37. What other prescription (nonhypertension) medications are you currently taking?	Other meds. for chronic conditions (e.g., arthritis, allergies, headaches)	_____
	Other meds. for temp. conditions (e.g., cold, flu, etc.)	_____

Table 3-3. Exercise

List the kinds of exercise that you regularly get:

Exercise	Times/Week
_____	_____
_____	_____
_____	_____

Do you feel that you get enough exercise? Yes _____ No _____
Has a physician ever told you not to do certain exercises? Yes _____ No _____
   If yes, explain _____
Do you have any physical problems that would keep you from exercising?
   Yes _____ No _____
Would you be interested in starting a regular exercise program?
   Yes _____ No _____
How physically active do you consider yourself to be?

Very active	Active	Average	Inactive	Very inactive
1	2	3	4	5

Were there periods in your adult life when you were more physically active than you are now?
   Yes _____ No _____
Have you ever tried to start a walking, jogging/running or cycling program and not stuck with it? Yes _____ No _____. If yes, complete the following:
a) Approximately how far or for how long were you *walking/running/cycling?*
                                                  (circle one)
                        _____ miles _____ minutes
b) Number of times per week: 1   2   3   4   5   6   7   (circle one)
c) How enjoyable was this activity?

Very enjoyable	Enjoyable	Neutral	Unenjoyable	Very unenjoyable
1	2	3	4	5

d) Reason(s) for discontinuing: _____

Have you ever attempted to start a regular exercise program (other than walking, running, or cycling) and not stuck with it: Yes _____ No _____

Attempt #	Exercise(s)	Alone or with others?	For how long?	Reason discontinuing
1.				
2.				
3.				
4.				
5.				
6.				

Do any friends or family members exercise regularly? (At least 3 times per week)
   Yes _____ No _____ If yes, complete the following:

Name/Relationship	Type of exercise
1.	
2.	
3.	

Have you ever had an exercise-related injury in your adult life? Yes _____ No _____ If Yes, complete the following:

Nature of injury	Date of injury	Activity	Treatment	Downtime
1.				
2.				
3.				
4.				

Do you currently have any medical problems that might interfere with your participation in an exercise program? Yes _____ No _____

Table 3-4. Diet

How much do you weigh now? _____
Weight history:
How long have you been at this weight (plus or minus 5 pounds) ____ years
Weight during childhood: ____ Underweight or normal ____ Overweight
Weight during adolescence: ____ Underweight or normal ____ Overweight
If you are overweight now, when was the last time you were at a normal weight? ____
Have you tried to lose weight before? Yes ____   No ____

Method	Date(s)	Amount of weight loss

Have you tried to make any other changes in your diet for health reasons?
    Yes ____   No ____
If yes, what changes _____
Are you trying to follow any kind of diet now?
    ____ No diet   ____ Physician-prescribed diet
    ____ Self-prescribed diet
    If yes, what kind of diet _____
    When did you begin this diet _____
    What percent of time do you actually follow your diet? _____
List all of the foods that you ate today and yesterday:
Breakfast: _____   Breakfast: _____
Snack: _____   Snack: _____
Lunch: _____   Lunch: _____
Snack: _____   Snack: _____
Dinner: _____   Dinner: _____
Snack: _____   Snack: _____
Typical Weekly Eating Pattern
(Indicate how many days per week each meal or snack is eaten in each situation.)

	Home	Brown-bag	Restaurant/ cafeteria	Fast food	Other
Morning meal					
Snack					
Lunch					
Snack					
Dinner					
Snack					

Is anyone else in the household on a special diet? _____
Who usually prepares the food eaten at home? _____
Who buys the groceries? _____
What kind of food is available at work? _____
    Is it possible to bring a brown-bag lunch? _____
Do you add salt to food? ____ None ____ At the table ____ In cooking
    If yes, ____ Light ____ Moderate ____ Heavy
How often do you drink alcoholic beverages?

Type	Amount	How often

Mark each of the following statements with a Y if it is true about you or a N if it is not true.
____ I eat fast most of the time.
____ I hardly notice what I eat.
____ I weigh myself at least once a week.
____ I like to eat sweets.
____ I like to eat chips, pretzels, nuts, or other salty snacks.
____ I am very aware of my weight and/or what I eat.
____ I like to reward myself with food.
____ I often eat when I am not really hungry.
____ I eat 3 meals each day.
____ I overeat when I am emotionally upset.

Table 3-5. Smoking

Have you ever smoked or used tobacco? Yes _____ No _____
   Type: (circle one) Cigarettes   Cigar   Pipe   Chew
Number of cigarettes/day _____ How many years at this rate? _____
How many years total smoking? _____ Want to quit or cut down? Yes _____ No _____
Former: Smoked _____ cigarettes per day for _____ years.
Brands:_____
When did you quit? _____ Why? _____

learn of possible barriers to implementing such a program. Table 3–4 is a very cursory screening for possible dietary interventions.

MEASUREMENT OF BLOOD PRESSURE

The primary measure of outcome in the nonpharmacological treatment of hypertension is the patient's blood pressure. Unlike many other psychophysiological disorders, such as headache or irritable bowel syndrome, for which one must rely heavily on the patient's self-report to determine if treatment is succeeding, in hypertension treatment the outcome is readily observable by the patient and the therapist.

As pointed out in Chapter 2, the autoregulation of BP is a highly complex physiological business; there are many factors which affect it. Likewise, because of the potential lability of this response, there are many factors that affect its measurement. *A key to evaluating treatment outcome is a well-standardized set of procedures for measuring BP*. We cannot emphasize this enough. The procedures for measuring BP in the therapist's office should be as standardized as is feasible. With standardized measurement, the therapist and the patient will know if treatment is having the desired effect on BP.

Because BP, by its very nature, is a continually changing response, alternating between the momentary peak of systolic pressure and the quiescent resting value of diastolic pressure, and because all measurement of BP other than by continuous recording from an arterial cannula is an approximation, we will, in this chapter, recommend some standard procedures for measuring BP in the clinical setting. We also provide a few comments about home BPs and 24-hour ambulatory BPs.

Measurement of Blood Pressure in the Clinic

The standard way of measuring BP is by means of auscultation. One uses an inflatable cuff to block or occlude the flow of arterial blood in the arm, and then slowly releases the pressure, listening with a stethoscope over the artery distally (downstream) of the cuff for the characteristic sounds that occur as blood begins to flow through the occluded artery.

We define systolic BP as that pressure at which one can just begin to detect sounds of blood flow in the occluded artery. This represents the peak pressure in the artery at each contraction of the heart. By like fashion, we usually define diastolic BP as the pressure at which all sounds disappear (5th phase). These distinctive sounds, named after the physician (Korotkoff), who elucidated their meaning, are the key to obtaining BP. Diastolic BP represents the lowest pressure in the artery, between heartbeats.

The pressures required in the cuff are usually measured in units of millimeters of mercury (mm Hg). In fact, pressure represents the force required on a specified area to sustain a column of mercury measuring so many millimeters high.

The standard device to measure BP is thus a mercury manometer and an occluding cuff. If, as a therapist, you are planning to see many hypertensive patients, it might be well to invest in a mercury sphygmomanometer. They are about $80 at medical supply houses.

An alternative in common use is the aneroid manometer. It is a spring-loaded pressure gauge calibrated to give a dial reading equivalent to millimeters of mercury. These devices can easily get out of calibration and should be checked against a mercury column every 3 months or so.

Another device of growing popularity is the sphygmomanometer in which the SBP and DBP are detected by an electronic microphone and circuit, which then display the SBP and DBP on a digital readout. This certainly eliminates the human judgment problem and the ear-eye coordination required in standard auscultation. However, the devices tend to underestimate systolic BP and overestimate diastolic BP slightly (Kaplan, 1986).

Standardized Measurement Conditions

We would recommend the following standardized measurement conditions:

1. The patient should be seated in a straightback chair with the feet on the floor. The patient should sit quietly for at least 5 minutes prior to taking the first BP reading. Ten minutes would probably be better. If the patient has just arrived in the office or clinic, we recommend allowing at least 5 minutes of being seated before beginning the assessment described above.

2. Pressure can be taken from either arm, but the same arm should be used consistently. There can easily be a 5–10 mm Hg difference between the two arms. We recommend the nondominant arm. At an initial visit, BP should be measured in both arms. If there is a noticeable difference, say more than 5 mm Hg, then the arm with the higher pressure should be used on all subsequent visits.
3. The BP cuff should be at the level of the heart. Thus, the arm on which the cuff is placed should be supported at the elbow by a firm surface.
4. Pump up the pressure in the cuff rapidly to a value about 20 mm Hg above what you suspect systolic BP will be. Then bleed the pressure down at a constant rate. Do *not* stop the bleed down between systolic BP and diastolic BP. Also, be sure to reduce the pressure fully between readings.
5. Avoid talking with the patient while determining BP. The mere act of speaking, on even a neutral subject, can raise BP by 10 mm Hg or more.
6. We recommend taking 3 measurements at each visit with about 2 minutes between measurements. One can either average all 3 values or discard the first and average the last 2.
7. We strongly recommend scheduling visits at which BP is to be taken at the same time of day. There is sizeable diurnal variation in BP (see, Kaplan, 1986), which could mislead the therapist and the patient.

Caveats

BP can show marked changes with changes in posture. For example, data from our laboratory show a 10 mm Hg difference (increase) in DBP from supine position to standing erect.

If you routinely have the patient sit in a recliner (as is commonly the case in many of the stress-management procedures), and have the patient's feet supported by the footrest, as opposed to being on the floor, such a postural change can decrease BP by about 5 mm Hg.

As a matter of routine, one should probably take radial pulse rate at the same time BP is measured. This measure of heart rate (HR) can provide valuable data for both stress management and exercise treatments.

It is important that the cuff itself be the correct size. (Technically, it is the size of the inflatable bladder within the cuff that counts; the bladder size tends to vary with the size of the cuff.) For individuals with very large upper arms, either due to muscle development or more likely to being very overweight, the standard-sized cuff is not large enough. A wider cuff, known in some circles as a "thigh cuff," is usually available and should be used.

Office Hypertension

A phenomenon that has been observed clinically for many years is so-called *office hypertension*. By this term is meant that some individuals show elevated BP in the physician's office but not in other settings (Kaplan, 1986). It has been known for some time (Mancia et al., 1983), and recently documented in 24-hour ambulatory-BP-monitoring studies (Pickering et al., 1982), that the highest average BP across the entire 24-hour day is found in the physician's office.

We suspect that the therapist who delivers nonpharmacological therapy would see the same phenomenon in the office, although this is not known for certain. One of us recently conducted a study of this phenomenon (Gerardi, Blanchard, Andrasik, & McCoy, 1985): A series of 40 medicated hypertensives had been taught to measure their BP at home (see next section). The average BP at home for 1 week was compared to BPs determined in the physician's office. We arbitrarily called patients *office hypertensives* or *office responders* if the office BP exceeded the home BP by 10 mm Hg; they constituted 32.5% of the sample. Likewise, we identified a subset of 10 patients (25%) whose home BPs exceeded office BPs by 10 mm Hg. They were termed *home responders*.

We compared the three groups on a number of psychological tests and to our surprise found no differences among the three groups on measures of anxiety (STAI [Spielberger, Gorsuch, & Lushene, 1970] state or trait, SCL-90-Anxiety) or depression (BDI [Beck et al., 1961] SCL-90-Depression). However, the middle group (nonresponders) were more hostile (SCL-90) and angry (trait anger) than either of the other two groups.

We have also tentatively identified a way to detect office hypertensives. If one measures BP under resting conditions and then subjects the patient to the mild mental stress of performing arithmetic in the head and reporting the answer (we have the patient count aloud from 30 to 0 by 3s and then from 100 to 0 by 7s) and again measures BP, one will undoubtedly find a rise in BP. For us, 9 of 13 office hypertensives had an increase in SBP of 10 mm Hg or greater. Thus, a rise of 10 mm or more should at least make one suspicious.

One might next raise the question of whether to treat patients who are hypertensive only when they are measured in the office. Our view is that one should provide treatment to these patients for the simple reason that all of the risk-factor data and studies discussed in Chapter 1 are based on sitting office pressures. Thus, the patients with BP elevated in the physician's office are at increased risk for heart attack or stroke, regardless of their home BPs.

Home Blood Pressures

One of us (EBB) has for the last 5 years routinely asked patients to monitor and report BPs taken at home on a daily basis. There is some evidence (Kleinhart et al., 1984) that home BPs are more representative of 24-hour ambulatory BPs than office BPs and are better predictors of serious cardiovascular illness than are office BPs.

On a clinical level, home BPs present a potential advantage and a potential detriment (which probably can be overcome). The advantages of home BPs are they keep the patient focused on the nonpharmacological treatment program by serving as a daily reminder to relax, exercise, or count calories. Moreover, as the patient's BP begins to decrease, this "hard evidence" can be very reinforcing to the patient to stay with the therapy.

On the other hand, this focusing of attention could backfire and make the patient a bit overconcerned (almost "neurotic") about BP. Moreover, because the changes in BP may be a bit slow (weeks to months), this might discourage the patient.

Clinical tip. It is important to forewarn the patient that any nonpharmacological treatment will be relatively slow—certainly taking weeks to months to show the size decrease in BP that one might see in days to a couple of weeks with drugs. This forewarning may prevent early discouragement and subsequent early termination.

Some number of patients will already own a sphygmomanometer. For those who do not, most should easily be able to afford an aneroid sphygmomanometer for measuring BP at home. There are several on the market that come with a built-in stethoscope that sell for from $20 to $30. There are also available electronic sphygmomanometers that give a digital readout of SBP and DBP. These are a bit more expensive, costing from $50 to $100. Their advantage is that the patient does not have to learn to detect the Korotkoff sounds and master the eye-ear coordination task. It is helpful if you have the information available to tell the patient to purchase the sphygmomanometer.

Once the patient has purchased the sphygmomanometer, have the patient bring it to the office for instruction in its use. (We have had patients who, on their own without training, begin using them with the stethoscope on the proximal rather than distal side of the cuff.) A dual stethoscope is useful for this instruction so that the patient can grow accustomed, under supervision, to detecting the onset of Korotkoff sounds (SBP) the muffling associated with the 4th phase, and the offset associated with the 5th phase (the usual definition of DBP).

Stress to the patient the necessity of taking BP at home at essentially the same time of day and under the same conditions. We would suggest having the patient record the home BPs and returning the readings to you on a regular basis—say at each visit.

Our reason for preferring the nondominant arm for clinic BPs is that the patient will probably take his own pressures in the nondominant arm because it is easier to manipulate the pressure-release valve with the dominant hand.

Twenty-four Hour Ambulatory Monitoring of BP

It appears that within *research* on nonpharmacological treatment of BP, we are rapidly moving to the use of the 24-hour ambulatory BP record as the "gold standard" for determining treatment effects. The advent of reasonably reliable 24-hour BP recording devices (Kaplan, 1986) has sparked this interest. These devices are still very expensive (about $7,500 for 24-hour recording unit to be worn by the patient and base unit to decode the stored values from the RAM pack). We would not recommend them for routine clinical practice. The fee in some places for a 24-hour record on a clinical basis is $200 to $300.

Recent research by Pickering and his colleagues (Pickering et al., 1982, 1985) with the 24-hour ambulatory monitor has confirmed that BP may well be highest either in the physician's office or at work. The 24-hour record may be especially useful with so-called labile hypertension in terms of identifying the range of pressures and to some extent the situations most frequently associated with elevated pressures.

There are now good data to support the fact that the 24-hour ambulatory BP record is more highly correlated with later morbidity and mortality than are simple office pressures (Perloff, Sokolow, & Cowan, 1983).

PSYCHOLOGICAL TESTING AND HYPERTENSION

Hypertension has a history of being considered a classical psychosomatic disorder (Alexander, 1939, 1950; Davies, 1971). The early anecdotal work (summarized by Weiner, 1977) depicted the hypertensive primarily as having difficulties "about the expression of hostility, aggression, resentment, rage, rebellion, ambition or dependency." (p. 124). More recent psychosomatic theorizing and research have focused on the possible roles of anger and hostility in essential hypertension (Diamond, 1982), and particularly on the inability of hypertensives to adequately express these emotions.

There has also been long standing interest in so-called neurogenic hypertension (DeQuattro & Miura, 1973; Esler, Julius, Zweifler, Randall, Harburg, Gardiner, & DeQuattro, 1977) and the related notion that chronic anxiety and anger could lead to hypertension by way of excessive sympathetic nervous system tone. In one elegant study, Whitehead, Blackwell, DeSilva and Robinson (1977) had hypertensive patients measure BP four times daily and simultaneously rate their degree of anxiety and anger on visual analog scales over a 7-week period. There were significant within-subject correlations, the highest being between SBP and anxiety (median $r = 0.36$).

In the work at one of our laboratories (EBB) we have routinely administered a number of standard psychological tests to hypertensive patients during the initial assessment. Our impression is that, as a group, hypertensive patients are less psychologically distressed than are patients with other stress-related disorders such as headache or irritable bowel syndrome. One preliminary study from our laboratory (Acerra, Andrasik, Blanchard, Appelbaum, Fletcher, & McCoy, 1983) tended to confirm this suspicion.

Nevertheless, in the interest of providing a comprehensive view of the hypertensive patient and as much useful information as possible, we present below the psychological test norms on a sample of about 100 hypertensive patients.

Psychological Test Norms for Hypertension

The sample on which the data to be presented below was gathered consisted of 103 hypertensives (72 male, 31 female of average age 48.6 [range 27 to 65]); 68 were on two antihypertensive medications at the time of the testing, while the other 35 were on no medications.

The psychological test battery included:

Beck Depression Inventory (Beck et al., 1961);
State-Trait Anxiety Inventory (Spielberger, Gorsuch, & Lushene, 1970);
State-Trait Anger Scale (Spielberger, 1980);
Buss-Durkee Scale (a measure of hostility) (Buss & Durkee, 1957);
Jenkins Activity Survey (for Type A behavior) (Jenkins, Zyzanski, & Roserman, 1965);
Social Readjustment Rating Scale (for life events) (Holmes & Rahe, 1967).

In Table 3–6 below, in addition to the normative data, we include the median scores on selected tests from a group of 68 paid volunteers who went through much of the testing. They were comprised of 19 males and 49 females, of mean age 41.7, range 21 to 68 who were relatively free of all psychosomatic symptoms. In Table 3–7 are normative data on our

Table 3-6. Psychological Test Norms for Hypertensives

| Beck Depression Inventory | | State-Trait Anxiety | | | |
| | | State | | Trait | |
Scores	Cumulative frequency (%)	Scores	Cumulative frequency (%)	Scores	Cumulative frequency (%)
0–2	43.6	20–24	17.5	20–24	7.3
3–5	63.4	25–29	42.3	25–29	21.9
6–8	74.3	30–40	58.8	30–34	41.7
9–11	92.1	35–39	77.3	35–39	65.6
12–14	97.0	40–44	87.6	40–44	80.2
15–17	100.0	45–49	94.8	45–49	93.8
		50+	100.0	50+	100.0
n	101	n	97	n	96
Median	3	Median	31	Median	36
Mean	4.6	Mean	33.5	Mean	36.7
Median score of normal controls	3	Median score of normal controls	30	Median score of normal controls	33

| Rathus Assertiveness Scale | | Social Readjustment Rating Scale (Life Events) | |
Scores	Cumulative frequency (%)	Scores	Cumulative frequency (%)
−40 or less	4.3	0–40	17.5
−30−−39	9.7	41–80	29.9
−20−−29	15.1	81–120	47.4
−10−−19	24.7	121–160	61.9
0−−9	38.7	161–200	77.3
+1−10	46.2	201–240	89.7
11−20	59.1	241–280	92.8
21−30	81.7	281–320	96.9
31−40	91.4	321	100.0
41+	100	n	97
n	93	Median	124
Median	+12		
Mean	9.2	Mean	134.9
Median score of normal controls	+9	Median score of normal controls	120

Table 3-7. Psychological Test Norms for Hypertension

| | State-Trait Anger Scale | | |
| | State | | Trait |
Scores	Cumulative frequency (%)	Scores	Cumulative frequency (%)
15	76.6	15–19	10.1
16–20	92.6	20–24	32.6
21–25	95.7	25–29	71.9
26–30	95.7	30–34	84.3
31–35	97.9	35–39	96.6
36	100.0	40	100.0
n	94	n	89
Median	15	Median	28
Mean	16.5	Mean	27.7

Table 3-7. (Continued)

Jenkins Activity Survey

Total		Speed & Impatience		Job Involvement		Hard Driving & Competitive	
Scores	Cumulative frequency (%)	Scores	Cumulative frequency (%)	Scores	Cumulative frequency (%)	Scores	Cumulative frequency (%)
80–119	5.1	36–119	22.2	80–119	1.1	39–79	10.1
120–159	20.4	120–159	43.4	120–159	21.1	80–119	54.5
160–199	44.9	160–199	65.7	160–199	43.3	120–159	96.0
200–239	56.1	200–239	80.8	200–239	75.6	160–199	100.0
240–279	73.5	240–279	89.9	240–279	94.4		
280–319	92.9	280–319	94.9	280–319	97.8		
320	100.0	320	100.0	320	100.0		
n	98	n	99	n	90	n	99
Median	208	Median	167	Median	213	Median	117
Mean	223	Mean	180	Mean	206	Mean	113

Buss-Durkee Hostility Scale

Total		Anger		Irritability		Guilt	
Scores	Cumulative frequency (%)	Scores	Cumulative frequency (%)	Scores	Cumulative frequency (%)	Scores	Cumulative frequency (%)
0–9	3.2	0–1	34.4	0–1	9.7	0–1	34.4
10–19	23.7	2–3	62.4	2–3	30.1	2–3	64.5
20–29	58.1	4–5	84.9	4–5	58.1	4–5	91.4
30–39	88.2	6–7	97.8	6–7	79.6	6–7	98.9
40–49	100.0	8–9	100.0	8–10	100.0	8	100.0
n	93	n	93	n	93	n	93
Median	28	Median	3	Median	5	Median	3
Mean	26.8	Mean	3.0	Mean	5.0	Mean	2.7

hypertensives for psychological tests for which we do not have comparison data from the group of paid normal volunteers.

As one can tell from the data in Table 3–6, and to some degree from Table 3–7, our hypertensives are a fairly "normal" group in terms of psychological tests.

This finding has two important implications: (1) one would not ordinarily expect to see much elevation or deviation on psychological tests taken by the hypertensive patient. If one then finds deviations, it is perhaps more significant than if found in a headache patient (because it is more out of the ordinary) and thus should be attended to. It may be that the psychological disturbance is not related to the hypertension. However, if one is treating the "whole patient" (see Chapter 9) one should then attend to these aberrant findings.

Second, it is known that severe life stress can lead to transient elevations in BP (Weiner, 1977). Thus, finding a very high score (say about 240 based on Table 3–6) on the life events measure should lead one to consider doing nothing other than waiting, since BP might return to the normal range on its own with time.

Finally, the data in Table 3–7 from Spielberger's State-Trait Anger Scale do provide indirect support for the role of unexpressed anger in hypertension. Over three quarters of our sample (76.6%) deny any feelings of anger at the time of the assessment (State-Anger), yet the level of Trait Anger is, on average, at a moderate level (median score of 28). Of course, because we have no way of knowing if this basal level of anger is, in fact, expressed under appropriate provocation, this remains at best speculative.

Chapter 4

Stress Management: Relaxation Therapies

OVERVIEW

There are a variety of psychological treatment procedures—primarily biofeedback and relaxation training, but sometimes including assertiveness training, time-management skills, elements of cognitive therapy, and general supportive psychotherapy—that have come to be subsumed under the term *Stress Management*. As an aside, it is our impression that there is a great deal of so-called stress management marketed but little systematic research on it. In fact, there is far from universal agreement as to what is included in stress management and, equally as important, what is *not* included.

Nevertheless, over the past few years in the field of nonpharmacological treatment of hypertension, most of the more psychological treatments (as contrasted to dietary interventions and exercise) have been lumped under the term *Stress Management* (e.g., McCaffrey & Blanchard, 1985). We shall follow this evolving usage in this book.

As noted in the Acknowledgments, one of us (EBB) has been involved in this line of research and practice for almost 15 years. Accordingly, it is primarily his view of this field and his treatment procedures that are described. For this reason, Stress Management in this book will refer only to various forms of biofeedback and various forms of relaxation training. None of the other procedures listed at the top of this page have been utilized systematically. Thus, in keeping with our goal of describing assessment and treatment procedures evaluated in our respective laboratories and clinics, only biofeedback and relaxation are described in this chapter.

41

Rationale

Somewhat different rationales have been advanced for the different Stress Management techniques. For Relaxation Training, it has been assumed that an increased overall level of arousal, manifested by some combination of increased muscle tension and/or increased sympathetic nervous system activity, was responsible for elevated BP (Patel, 1977; Benson, 1975; Agras, Taylor, Kraemer, Allen, & Schneider, 1980). It then follows that techniques that decrease overall arousal, and its various manifestations in the striate musculature and sympathetic activation, should lead to a decrease in elevated BP. This assumption, often more implicit than explicit, has been challenged in part by Julius and his colleagues (Weder & Julius, 1985). Moreover, this assumption has been tested explicitly in only a few of the many treatment studies.

The techniques that reduce arousal are thought to operate either primarily through reduced skeletal muscle tension levels (the progressive muscle relaxation of Jacobson [1938] and its variants, and EMG [electromyogram] biofeedback) or through decreasing peripheral sympathetic nervous system tone (thermal biofeedback [Fahrion et al., 1986], electrodermal biofeedback [Patel, 1973] or autogenic training), or through some combination of the two, such as the meditation or passive relaxation as popularized by Benson (1975).

The other form of Stress Management, direct biofeedback of blood pressure (Shapiro, 1974), has been assumed to work directly on the peripheral vascular system and to bring about reductions in BP.

Thus, although some forms of biofeedback (thermal, EMG) could be seen as belonging conceptually with Relaxation Training, for convenience and because of methodological and implementation issues, we will consider all forms of biofeedback together in Chapter 5 and all forms of relaxation training together in this chapter.

RELAXATION TRAINING

The oldest class, or category, of the stress management techniques used with hypertension are various forms of relaxation training; the oldest form of relaxation training which has been used to treat hypertension is Progressive Muscle Relaxation, developed by Edmund Jacobson (1938). As far back as 1936 Jacobson was reporting sizeable decreases in BP accompanying deeply relaxed states. In the 1970s Herbert Benson (1975) investigated and popularized an alternative form of relaxation he called the "Relaxation Response." A third form of relaxation training is Autogenic Training, popularized by Schultz and Luthe (1969). Although widely used in Europe (and in recent years in the Soviet Union), its use is still not widespread in this country. One of us (EBB) has used all three of these forms of relaxation in various experimental studies.

In this section of Chapter 4, we shall describe each of these three forms of relaxation. Each subsection will include (a) a brief overview of the literature supporting the efficacy of the particular technique in treating hypertension; (b) a brief summary of the authors' own experience in using the technique; (c) detailed descriptions of the relaxation procedures themselves; (d) clinical hints and findings from the literature that pertain to treatment methodology (e.g., value of home practice, etc.).

PROGRESSIVE MUSCLE RELAXATION

Almost no one today utilizes true Progressive Muscle Relaxation (PMR) in the lengthy and laborious form advocated by Jacobson (1938). Instead, various forms of abbreviated Progressive Muscle Relaxation, popularized by Wolpe (1958) and Paul (1966), and utilizing 4 to 12 training sessions spread over 4 to 8 weeks have become the norm.

The Stanford studies. Although there were small scale reports on the use of abbreviated PMR in the literature in the early 1970s, the most influential report was that of Agras and his colleagues (Taylor, Farquhar, Nelson, & Agras, 1977). Thirty-one patients (23 male, 8 female, average age 48.2), who were undergoing routine medical care (including medication) for their essential hypertension, were randomized to: (a) abbreviated PMR administered live on an individual basis; (b) supportive psychotherapy aimed at helping patients to identify tension producing situations and to plan ways to handle them; (c) continued BP monitoring in the hypertension clinic. All three groups continued to receive standard medical care for their hypertension. All BPs were measured in the medical care setting, thus assuring that the nurse making the measurement was "blind" to treatment condition. The therapist was also kept blind to BP values from the assessments. From 5 to 6 sessions of approximately 30 minutes in duration were held in the relaxation condition and in the supportive therapy condition. Nine patients dropped out.

Results at the end of 8 weeks showed the relaxation group had significantly greater decreases in SBP and DBP than did either the supportive therapy group or the continued medical care group, which did not differ significantly from each other. The relaxation group showed an average decrease in BP of 13.6/4.9 mm Hg. At a 6-month follow-up the reductions in BP for the relaxation treatment were maintained. However, improvement in the other two groups (probably due to medication changes), led to there being no significant difference among the groups at follow-up.

An interesting aspect of the study reported by the authors was that the five relaxation patients whose BPs had been poorly controlled on medication at the start of training (>140/90) showed the most improvement (−21/−12 mm Hg).

This study, which contained control features absent in all previous reports, seemed to establish that abbreviated PMR with regular home practice could lead to clinically meaningful reductions in BP and that the effects were specific to the treatment rather than due to nonspecific attentional factors.

Agras and his colleagues continued their studies of abbreviated PMR with several additional controlled-trials: Brauer, Horlick, Nelson, Farquhar, and Agras (1979) compared (a) 10 weekly sessions of individually administered PMR in which patients received a tape to assist home practice to (b) a 10-week program of largely home-based, self-administered PMR and (c) 10 weekly sessions of individual nondirective counseling dealing with stress and tension in the patients' lives. The home-based patients were seen for initial relaxation training sessions and then had practice guided by a series of audiotapes containing the same information as was given in (a).

Although the office-based treatment showed substantial decreases in BP (11.0/6.1 mm Hg) at end of treatment, the changes were not significantly greater than those in the other two conditions. At a 6-month follow-up, however, the individual office-based treatment was significantly superior to both of the other two conditions (−18/−10), which did not differ. The minimal-contact home-based treatment was largely ineffective (+1/−4 mm Hg at 6-month follow-up).

The last major study (Southam, Agras, Taylor, & Kraemer, 1982; Agras, Southam, & Taylor, 1983) involved patients obtained from a worksite screening program who were assessed both at the clinic and the worksite, including ambulatory BP monitoring at the worksite. The treatment consisted of 8 weekly half-hour training sessions in PMR with daily home practice. A set of 3 audiotapes was given to the experimental patients to guide home practice. Nineteen patients received the relaxation training, while 23 patients in the control condition had BP periodically assessed. At end of treatment the PMR group had significantly greater decreases in BP at the worksite (7.8/4.6 mm Hg) and for DBP in the clinic (12.6 mm Hg). At a 6-month follow-up the PMR group had significantly lower DBPs. A 15-month follow-up (Agras et al., 1983) on 30 patients (12 experimental, 18 controls) revealed no significant between-group differences. However, the experimental groups' DBPs were still significantly reduced at the clinic (−13.8) and at the worksite (−7.4) and, in fact, were slightly lower than end of treatment values.

Summary. Taken as a whole, this series of studies provide fairly strong evidence for the efficacy of individually administered, abbreviated PMR combined with audiotape assisted, regular home practice. The initial decreases in BP for this treatment across the three studies were: −13.6/−4.9; −11.0/−6.1; −11.7/−12.6. In follow-ups of 6 to 15 months the reductions had been fairly well maintained. Mild improvements in control conditions and the inherent variability in the data frequently prevented the decreases from being statistically better than the controls. Other studies (e.g., Hatch, Klatt, Supik, Rios, Fisher, Bauer, & Shimotsu, 1985) have generally confirmed the findings of the Agras group.

Results of PMR by the Present Authors

Our first study (Blanchard, Murphy, Haynes, & Abel, 1979) involving PMR was a small-scale comparison of several relaxation techniques. Eight patients (4 medicated, 4 nonmedicated), whose DBPs remained above 90 mm Hg across 4 baseline screening sessions, received 12 individually administered training sessions in PMR over a 6-week period of time. Regular home practice was expected and a handout (but no audiotape) was provided to assist the practice.

The BP values (sitting, after 10 minutes of rest) for these 8 patients from baseline, end-of-treatment, and a 3-month follow-up are given in Table 4–1.

Initial results were very poor with an 8.6 mm Hg *rise* in SBP and a 3.6 mm Hg decrease in DBP. At three months, our results were

Table 4-1. Authors' BP Results from Abbreviated
Progressive Muscle Relaxation

	Baseline	1 week Posttreatment	3 months Posttreatment
SBP	156.0	164.6	151.0
DBP	95.7	92.1	88.7

comparable to those of other investigators: a 5.0 mm Hg decrease in SBP and a clinically significant 7.0 mm Hg decrease in DBP.

The second study (Blanchard et al., 1986) was a more elaborate effort: A controlled comparison of abbreviated PMR with thermal biofeedback in the treatment of patients whose BP was, at the beginning of the study, controlled (<140/90) on two antihypertensive medications. Of 43 patients (24 male, 19 female, average age 48.5) initially randomized to the abbreviated PMR condition, 34 finished treatment.

In this study, approximately half the patients were scheduled to be treated while on the two drugs, whereas the others were removed from the sympathetically active drug before treatment. Because many of the patients in the latter condition could not be withdrawn from the drug prior to treatment (because of dangerous rises in BP or the onset of symptoms), these initial withdraw failures were restabilized on the two drugs and treated while they were on the two drugs.

This treatment regimen consisted of 8 individually administered sessions, spread over 8 weeks. An outline of the whole relaxation training regimen is contained in Table 4–2. Detailed, verbatim

Table 4-2. Short-Term Effects of Abbreviated Progressive Muscle Relaxation on Blood Pressure of Medicated Hypertensives

Condition	BP Measure	Pretreatment	Posttreatment	Within group t	p
Treated while on	Home BPs				
two drugs	Supine SBP	130.7	129.6	0.83	ns
($n = 22$)	Standing SBP	130.6	129.0	1.02	ns
	Supine DBP	80.6	80.4	0.24	ns
	Standing DBP	87.8	86.0	2.14	0.04
	Clinic BPs ($n = 12$) (seated)				
	SBP	140.3	139.4	0.19	ns
	DBP	88.7	85.7	1.11	ns
Treated after	Home BPs				
withdrawal of	Supine SBP	128.2	128.8	−0.40	ns
second-stage drug	Standing SBP	132.7	133.0	−0.34	ns
($n = 9$)	Supine DBP	80.9	80.8	0.10	ns
	Standing DBP	87.9	87.3	0.50	ns
	Clinic BPs ($n = 5$) (seated)				
	SBP	131.2	127.8	0.89	ns
	DBP	86.0	78.4	1.44	ns

instructions for conducting the abbreviated PMR are presented later in Table 4–5.

As is obvious from the material in Table 4–2, the relaxation regimen is very similar to that described by Bernstein and Borkovec (1973) and to that which we have previously described (Blanchard & Andrasik, 1985) for the treatment of chronic headache. (It is also very similar to the regimen used by Agras and his colleagues [personal communication].)

The effects of this treatment program on BP (Blanchard et al., 1986) are presented in Table 4–3.

As can be seen, with the exception of standing DBP for the patients treated while still on two drugs, and the seated clinic DBP for patients withdrawn before treatment, the effects were modest and nonsignificant. In the latter case, the 7.6 mm decrease in DBP, although not statistically significant, was sizeable. (A possible explanation for these modest effects on BPs can be found in the following discussion of the effect of baseline BP on treatment response.)

On our so-called clinical endpoint of whether the patient could be successfully maintained while off the second-stage drug, the results were fairly disappointing: Only 9 of 34 (26%) were successful approximately 2 months after the drugs had been withdrawn. Nevertheless, we believe that abbreviated PMR can be a valuable treatment for some hypertensives and the procedures should be in the armamentarium of the clinician.

Table 4-3. Relaxation Training Regimen

Week no.	Session no.	Content
1	1	Introduction and rationale; training with 16 muscle groups; instruction on home practice
1	2	Discuss home practice; training with 16 muscle groups; introduce imagery
2	3	Discuss home practice; training with 16 muscle groups; continue imagery
3	4	Discuss home practice; training with 8 muscle groups
4	5	Discuss home practice; training with 4 muscle groups; encourage use of relaxation in stressful situations
5	6	Discuss home practice; training with 4 muscle groups; relaxation by recall; instructions in breathing
6	7	Discuss home practice; training with 4 muscle groups; cue-controlled relaxation
7	No session	Patient practices at home
8	8	Check progress; cue-controlled relaxation

Baseline Effects on Hypertensives' Response to Relaxation Therapy

In a brilliant analysis of the literature on the use of relaxation therapies for hypertension, Jacob and his colleagues (Jacob, Kraemer, & Agras, 1977) plotted the effects of various forms of relaxation (that is, the group average decrease in BP) on a group basis as a function of the group's average BP at the beginning of treatment. They also made similar plots for the effects of placebo in double-blind, placebo-controlled drug trials. Simplified versions of this regression analysis are contained in Figure 4–1.

Jacob has thus assumed that all relaxation therapies are equivalent for the purposes of his analysis. Certainly some of our data (Blanchard, Murphy, et al., 1979) and that of others (e.g., Chesney, Black, Swan, & Ward, 1987) tends to confirm this assumption.

If one makes the assumption that the regression line can be used for individual patient prediction, great utility emerges from the Figure. One

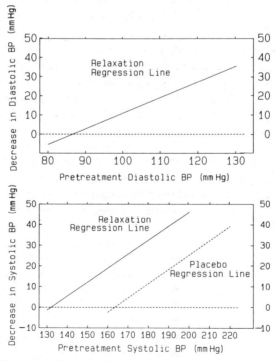

FIGURE 4–1. Effects of Relaxation Therapy as a Function of Average Beginning BP (redrawn from Jacob, Kraemer, & Agras, 1977)

can enter a starting, or initial, BP, either SBP or DBP, on the x axis and draw a vertical line up to the regression line; then moving to the left of the point of interception on the regression line, one can predict the amount of reduction in BP one would find for that patient. For example, if a patient presented with SBP of 160 mm Hg, one would predict a 17 mm decrease in SBP from relaxation therapy.

This regression analysis also provides a possible explanation of the very limited reductions in BP reported in Table 4–2. If one begins treatment with SBPs averaging only 130 mm of mercury, the regression line predicts essentially *zero* decrease in SBP from the relaxation training. This was what we found!

SUNY-AMC HYPERTENSION PROJECT RELAXATION TRAINING PROTOCOL

As we noted earlier, the abbreviated PMR program we use is modeled after that described by Bernstein and Borkovec (1973) in their book *Progressive Relaxation Training*. We provide a copy of this book to our therapists and ask them to study it. An outline of our training regimen is contained in Table 4–3.

Instructions for Relaxation Training

As you begin the relaxation training with your patients, there are several points to keep in mind. Remind them of the schedule of appointments for the relaxation training. This schedule consists of the patients being seen twice per week for Week 1, then once per week for Weeks 2, 3, 4, 5, and 6, then skipping a week and being seen once in Week 8. The first session lasts about 65 minutes. Tell the patient that later sessions will probably take about 30 to 40 minutes.

At each session it will be important to collect relaxation-practice diary sheets, to remind the patients to continue to send home BP measures to you to check to see how they are doing in general and to see if monitoring home BP has led them to discover anything about their hypertension, and to be supportive and empathic in order to maintain a good therapeutic relationship. *Only if the patients come to treatment can we help them; and only if they are involved enough to practice will we help them.*

Take the patient's blood pressure and pulse while the patient is in a reclined position. Then explain the treatment rationale as follows (you do not need to use this material verbatim):

> The form of treatment for hypertension we will begin today is known as progressive muscle relaxation training. This form of treatment has been successfully demonstrated by previous research to aid in controlling high blood pressure.

> Relaxation training consists of the systematic tensing and relaxing of the major muscle groups of the whole body. After going through this series of tension-release exercises or cycles, most people feel relaxed. With practice, and I want to emphasize the word *practice*, one can learn to become deeply relaxed fairly rapidly.

> Achieving a state of deep relaxation is a learned skill, somewhat like learning to ride a bicycle. To be really effective, one must practice regularly. Also as you practice, you should begin to be more aware of the tension in your body, to be able to recognize it earlier, and to localize it so that it becomes something you can more readily cope with.

> For this training to be of the most benefit to you, you should go through the exercises for about 20 minutes, twice per day. If you cannot find time for two practices per day, one practice is acceptable but not as good as twice per day. If you cannot, or will not, practice regularly, then you probably will not receive the major benefits of the training.

> Before we begin with the initial treatment session, let me briefly explain why relaxation training should help you to control your blood pressure.

> There are two parts to your nervous system: the *voluntary* part, which controls all of your movements and all of your senses; and the involuntary or *automatic* part of your nervous system, which regulates most of your bodily responses, such as how fast your heart beats, the level of your blood pressure, and so forth.

> This *automatic* part of your nervous system is called the *autonomic nervous system*. One of its main parts is called the *sympathetic nervous system*. It is involved in helping the body prepare for emergencies.

> One of your body's reactions to this so-called fight-or-flight response is increased muscle tension in many of the major muscles in your body. You may have noticed that when in a traffic jam, for example, your arms feel quite tense as you grip the wheel. Increased muscle tension, in turn, has the effect of "tightening down" on many of your blood vessels, specifically those that lead from your heart (that is, your arteries). Thus, these arteries become constricted and your blood pressure increases.

> Progressive muscle relaxation, then, is designed to help you to gain some degree of voluntary control over the autonomic, or automatic, nervous system by teaching you to recognize muscle tension and to employ a systematic technique to reduce it in your body, particularly when you are aroused for no adaptive reason.

> The reduced levels of muscle tension will subsequently induce a generalized state of relaxation, with correspondingly less constriction of blood vessels and lower blood pressure.

> Thus, we hope to be able to substitute a nondrug therapy for at least one of your drugs.

Next, pointing to the muscle groups on your body, show the patient the muscle groups that will be involved and demonstrate what you will want her or him to do. The reason for this, of course, is that the patients will have their eyes closed. You can make this point to them. The muscle groups will be:

hand and lower arm, right, left, then both together (have patient make a fist and tense lower arm)
upper arm, right, left, then both together (make a muscle)
lower leg and foot, right, left, then both together (foot up, pointed toward head)
thighs (press together)
abdomen (draw in)
chest and breathing (hold deep breath)
shoulders and lower neck (hunch shoulders up)
back of neck (press head against back of chair)
lips (press lips together without biting down)
eyes (squint)
lower forehead (frown, eyebrows down)
upper forehead (eyebrows up)

Tell the patient that you will want him to have his eyes closed during the entire training. Then, once the patient understands what the sequence will be, have the patient remove eyeglasses if he or she is wearing them, and have the patient take off very restrictive clothing such as jackets.

Go through the demonstration of the relaxation exercise using the right lower arm. In this you will ask the person to tense the right hand and lower arm, to attend to the sensations of tension in that arm, and then to relax it. (For most patients, when they relax the hand and arm, they will not relax the whole arm from the shoulder down.) Next, ask the patient to try again and when he or she relaxes, really let it go completely so that the whole arm from the shoulder all the way down can become limp. You can support the arm and show them what you mean. Repeat this until the patient seems to be able to let that arm become fairly relaxed, without catching it, as she relaxes on instruction.

Next, tell the patient that you will be instructing her to tense the various muscle groups you have mentioned, that you will be calling attention to the sensations she is probably experiencing and giving various other suggestions.

Next, go through the muscle groups as listed above. Have the patient tense the muscle group for 5 to 10 seconds, attend to the sensations of tension in that particular muscle group and area of the body; then relax the muscle, to notice the difference between the tension and the relaxation. For the limbs, you will do right lower arm and hand, then left lower arm and hand, and then the two together; right upper arm, left upper arm and the two together; right lower leg and foot, left lower leg and foot, and the two together. For all of the others you will not have this bilateral aspect. Between each muscle group, allow either about 20 seconds with perhaps a comment (e.g., "just continue to relax" or one of the between-exercise suggestions in the following section). This particular material is suggesting increased relaxation—which may help; use these suggestions after *every other* tension-release cycle and continue to cycle through the particular suggestions. There is no special magic to the particular wording, but try to use something approximating this content with which you also feel comfortable.

Go through the tension-relaxation exercises; this should probably take 20 minutes or so. At the end of all of the tension-relaxation cycles, go through the deepening exercise by counting from 1 to 5. (See following section on deepening after-tension-relaxation exercises.) Tell the person you are going to count from 1 to 5 and that as you count she will become more relaxed. Again interpolate suggestions of greater relaxation between the numbers and try to time the counts to an exhalation.

Once you have done the deepening suggestions, then ask the person to concentrate on breathing, to breathe through the nose, and to concentrate on breathing so that as the person breathes in, she can feel the cool air and as she exhales, she can feel the warm air. Finally, tell the patient to think the word *relax* as she exhales. Allow about 1 or 2 minutes for this and repeat the instructions at least once.

At this point you should fill out the Behavioral Relaxation Rating Scale (see Table 4–4).

After that, go through the reverse of the deepening counting from 5 back to 1. Tell the person that you are going to do that and suggest to her that, as you count, she is becoming more alert and at *two* will open her eyes, and at *one* will be back at a normal state of alertness.

Have the person remain seated after the alerting, but sitting up. Therefore, you want to drop the footrest so she is now in an upright seated position. Give back glasses to those who wear them. You want to inquire first if the patient became relaxed at all; secondly, if there were any particular signs of residual tension; third, if there were any other noticeable sensations or things to talk to you about. Obtain a self-rating of relaxation using the 1 (not relaxed) to 10 (very deeply relaxed) rating scale.

After this, give them the instruction sheet which repeats the muscle groups and the sequence. Also, ask the patient to record in a diary when she practiced, the length of time, and the approximate time of day. Have the patient try to scale how relaxed she became for each practice, using 1 as not being relaxed or tense and 10 as very deeply relaxed. You can also mention that many people are able to do this very readily but that some people need the assistance of a tape recording to help cue them. Give patients the audiotape for home practice and ask them to use it initially. Give patients a diary book and remind them to bring it to future sessions.

Verbatim Instructions During Tension-Relaxation Exercises

Now I want you to tense the muscles of your (*muscle area*) by (*tensing instructions*). Study the tensions located in (*tension location*). (*Pause*). Study those tensions.

(After subject has tensed the muscle group for 10 seconds):

Now *relax* the muscles of your (*muscle area*), and study the difference between the tension and the relaxation.

Between-exercise suggestions:

1. Just let yourself become more and more relaxed. If you feel yourself becoming drowsy that will be fine too. As you think of relaxation and of letting go of your muscles, they will become more loose . . . heavy . . . and relaxed. Just let your muscles go as you become more and more deeply relaxed.
2. (Pause 20 seconds.)
3. You are becoming more and more relaxed, drowsy and relaxed. As you become more relaxed you will feel yourself settling deep into the chair. All your muscles are becoming more and more comfortably relaxed . . . loose . . . heavy . . . and relaxed.
4. (Pause 20 seconds.)
5. The relaxation is growing deeper and still deeper. You are relaxed . . . drowsy and relaxed. Your breathing is regular and relaxed. With each breath you take in your relaxation increases, . . . and each time you exhale you spread the relaxation throughout your body.
6. (Pause 20 seconds.)
7. Note the pleasant feelings of warmth and heaviness that are coming into your body as your muscles relax completely. You will always be clearly aware of what you are doing and what I am saying as you become more deeply relaxed.
8. (Pause 20 seconds.)
9. Now the very deep state of relaxation is moving through all the areas of your body. You are becoming more and more comfortably relaxed . . . drowsy and relaxed. You can feel the comfortable sensations of relaxation as you go into a deeper . . . and deeper state of relaxation.
10. (Pause 20 seconds.)

Deepening After-Tension-Relaxation Exercises

Now I want you to relax all the muscles of your body; just let them become more and more relaxed. I am going to help you to achieve a deeper state of relaxation by counting from 1 to 5. As I count you will feel yourself becoming more and more deeply relaxed—. . . farther and farther down into a deep restful state of deep relaxation. One . . . you are going to become more deeply relaxed. Two . . . down, down into a very relaxed state. Three . . . four . . . more and more relaxed . . . *five*. *Deeply relaxed*.

Attention to Breathing

Now I want you to remain in your very relaxed state . . . I want you to begin to attend just to your breathing. Breathe through your nose. Notice the cool air as you breathe in (pair with inhalation) . . . and the warm moist air as you exhale (pair with exhalation) . . . . Just continue to attend to your breathing . . . . Now each time you exhale, mentally repeat the word *relax*. Inhale, exhale, *relax* (pair with respiratory cycle) . . . Inhale, exhale, *relax* . . . .

Procedures for Alerting

Now I am going to help you to return to your normal state of alertness. In a little while I shall begin counting backward from five to one. You will gradually become more alert. When I reach *two* I want you to open your eyes. When I get to *one* you will be entirely roused up in your normal state of alertness. Ready now? Five . . . four . . . you are becoming more and more alert. You feel very refreshed . . . three . . . *two* . . . Now your eyes are opened and you begin to feel very alert. Returning completely to your normal state . . . *one*. (Pause ten seconds.)

SECOND AND THIRD RELAXATION TRAINING SESSIONS

In addition to checking on the diary and how things have been going in general, you will want to inquire particularly as to success in doing the relaxation exercises. Check to see if patients noted the times in their diaries and made ratings of how relaxed they became. Inquire as to any difficulties and whether they seem to get relaxed. Also see if patients tried relaxing without the tape and how that went.

Next, you need to elicit from the person a pleasant, relaxing image or situation. Tell the patient that at the end of the exercises you will ask him or her to try to imagine this scene again, in order to help begin to pair some imaginal cues with the relaxed body state.

Go through the same set of exercises as you did before with the same kind of instructions. (You can omit the initial testing for the ability to relax the arm.) At the end of the exercises and the deepening, you should then describe to the patient the pleasant, relaxing image and ask the person to try to capture it in his or her mind's eye. Then do the alerting exercise. Again inquire at the end of it whether the patient became relaxed, if there were any residual tension sites, if there was difficulty attending to breathing, and if there had been any strange sensations. If a person is having some particular residual tension, the next time that you see him, you should probably do some additional tension-release cycles with the particular relevant muscle group if possible. Please note this in your progress note that goes into the chart.

Frequently patients will ask whether they should go through the exercises as a coping strategy when faced with stressful situations. You can leave this to their own discretion by telling them that they can try it and see if it helps. Tell them that as they become more proficient, they will learn to relax fairly deeply on a fairly rapid basis—and then they could certainly use it as a coping strategy. Tell them the more important thing would probably be to try to learn to relax as completely as possible and to practice the technique on a regular basis.

SESSION FOUR

The main purposes of this session are (a) to reduce the number of muscle groups the patient is using to achieve a state of deep relaxation, and (b) to continue to monitor the patient's progress.

It is hoped that it has become routine for you at each session to inquire (a) how things have been going in general for the patient; and (b) how the home practice of relaxation has been progressing, noting any problems, unusual occurrences, or side effects he may have had. You should also check and record the diary data on the patient's relaxation practice, and check to insure that the patient is continuing to send in his home BP measurements.

Tell patients to try to notice muscle tension as it begins and to see if they can ward if off by relaxing.

For Session 4, only 8 muscle groups will be used. See Bernstein and Borkovec's (1973) *Progressive Relaxation Training*, pages 33–34.

The groups we will use are (in order):

1. Both arms
2. Both lower legs
3. Abdomen
4. Chest (by deep breath)
5. Shoulders
6. Back of neck
7. Eyes
8. Forehead

For the lower arms have the patient hold both arms out, slightly flexed at the elbow, and tense the hands, lower arms, and upper arms.

Introduce this variation by telling the patient that you will be reducing the number of muscle groups as a step toward shortening the procedure and making it a tactic that is "more portable" and readily usable. Go through the muscle groups to be used and demonstrate the lower-arm flexion position.

Extend the interval between tension-relaxation cycles to at least 30 seconds.

At the end of the exercises, go through the "deepening by counting" procedure and then have the patient attend to breathing, and to mentally repeat the word *relax* as he exhales. Use the same instructions as before.

After alerting, inquire as to whether the patient was able to become deeply relaxed.

If there are any indications of problems, have the patient continue to use the longer procedure. If there were no problems, have the patient begin to use the shorter, eight-muscle-group procedure for home practice.

SESSION FIVE

In this session you will again be focusing on reducing the number of muscle groups used.

Of course, continue to monitor relaxation practice and record the diary information. Also remember to measure and record recumbent BP and pulse at the beginning and end of each session. For those who may not be doing too well, try to maintain their interest and enthusiasm. Also begin to direct the patient's attention to everyday events to see if the patient can begin to detect when he or she is becoming more tense through the day. Suggest that the person try to monitor this state and *begin to use the ability to relax as an active coping tactic*. By this you should suggest that the person try to become relaxed as he or she begins to feel tension, to try to catch the negative feelings early.

For Session 5, tell the patient that you will again be trying to shorten the exercises by going to only *four muscle groups*. These four groups are, in the order to use them: arms, chest, neck and shoulders, and face (especially eyes and forehead).

1. For the *arms*, use both arms together with closed fists and arms flexed slightly at the elbow.
2. For the *chest*, use the deep breath, which is held.
3. For the *neck*, have the patient hunch the shoulders slightly while drawing in and tensing the back of the neck.
4. For the *face*, have them close their eyes tightly while drawing up the rest of the face.

After demonstrating the four muscle groups, go through the tension-relaxation cycles with these four groups. Intersperse suggestions between each tension-release cycle. Then go through the deepening-by-counting exercise and the attention to breathing routine.

SESSIONS SIX AND SEVEN

At Session 6, especially inquire as to how practice has been since using the shorter procedure. If there have been special problems, proceed with the session as specified below but be sure to find out the source of the problems.

In this session you will introduce the notion of *Relaxation-by-Recall* and test to see how well the patient can handle this variation.

Introduce the idea by telling the patient again that one goal of the training is to be able to become relaxed readily and quickly in most situations as well as for the person to practice becoming relaxed on a daily basis. To help in the first goal, you are going to try something different: to see if the patient can become relaxed without going through the tension-relaxation cycle. Tell the patient you will be asking her or him to *recall* what the relaxed state felt like in her/his mind and to try to achieve that state without tensing the muscles.

Then run through the four muscle groups. Before starting, arrange for the patient to signal you, by raising a forefinger, if she has not been able to relax a particular muscle group. Ask patient (a) to focus attention on the muscles in the hands and arms; (b) very carefully identify any feelings or sensations of tension or tightness that might be present; especially focus on any tension feelings. (This should be spread over 10 to 15 seconds.)

Then ask the patient (a) to relax and to recall what it was like when she or he released the tension from that particular muscle group; (b) reemphasize having the patient relax, letting go of those particular muscles and allowing them to become more and more deeply relaxed. Allow 30 to 40 seconds to elapse (with the interjection of the usual suggestions).

Then ask patient to signal if the muscles are *not* deeply relaxed.

If she indicates they are *not* relaxed, try the same suggestions again.

If the patient indicates they are *still not* relaxed, then go through the actual tension-relaxation cycle.

If the patient indicates they are *relaxed*, go to the next muscle group.

For tensing *the chest* by using the deep breath, *do not use recall*. Use the actual breathing exercise.

At the end of relaxing the four muscle groups, take some time to focus on the breathing. Have the patient take a deep diaphragmatic breath and think the word *relax*, as she exhales. Repeat this several times. Now see if the patient is becoming relaxed to just the word.

Finally alert the patient. Then have him practice the deep breath in, conscious exhalation and saying to himself, "relax." This sets the stage for cue-controlled relaxation, which is formally introduced in Session 7. This concludes Session 6.

For Session 7, begin the session by asking about any difficulties in practicing the Relaxation-by-Recall at home.

Next, go through a 4-muscle-group relaxation induction using Relaxation-by-Recall as described above. After alerting the patient and having her or him practice the cue-controlled procedure, introduce the label by telling her this is the final step in reducing the relaxation training to a brief, portable procedure. Tell her it is called "Cue-Controlled Relaxation" and that it is designed for use throughout the day when she feels tense or wants to take a brief "relaxation break."

In addition to the regular practice, ask patients to use the cue-controlled procedure (several times per day). Suggest that they try it while riding to and from work, at work, at lunch and other times.

Remember the sequence is: (1) Take a deep breath; (2) consciously exhale; (3) let the shoulders consciously sag or slump, and (4) say to oneself, "relax." If convenient, the patient might close her eyes and relax a few moments after this brief exercise.

If the patient was *mostly* successful with recall, tell her to try recall at home but to be prepared to use the regular tension-relaxation cycles if she is not becoming relaxed.

If the patient was unsuccessful or only moderately successful, tell her not to be concerned, that it will come with practice and that she should stay with the regular tension relaxation cycles at the home practice.

SESSION EIGHT

1. At Session 8, check progress. Remind the patient that this is the last session for the relaxation training. Be sure to inquire as to the patient's general status.
2. Next, go through the four muscle group series using recall. Add actual tension-relaxation cycles if needed. Have the patient try to deepen the relaxation by mentally counting after you suggest this and then attend to his or her breathing. Let the patient remain relaxed for at least two minutes. Then alert the patient.
3. Review all of the procedures with the patient:
   a. 16 muscle groups
   b. 8 muscle groups
   c. 4 muscle groups
   d. relaxation-by-recall
   e. cue-controlled relaxation and its regular practice through the day
   f. use of relaxation as a coping strategy throughout the day
4. *EMPHASIZE:* a. the need for continued regular practice of the relaxation exercises
   b. the use of relaxation, especially cue-controlled relaxation, in the natural environment as an active coping strategy
   c. the need for continued records
5. Set up an appointment for a follow-up visit.

Transfer of Relaxation Effects to Everyday Activities

An obvious question a skeptic might raise about the value of relaxation training is whether the patient is merely learning to relax in the clinic (and at the physician's office) so that BP measurements taken there are artificially low—or do the effects of 20 to 30 minutes of relaxation training generalize to the patient's whole day in his natural environment? One way of addressing this question for yourself and for the patient is through the examination of home BP records. If these values show changes consistent with those seen in the clinic, they can be taken as evidence of generalization.

Fortunately, Agras and his colleagues have provided some good experimental evidence on this issue. In the studies cited earlier (Southam et al., 1982; Agras et al., 1983), there was evidence for statistically (and clinically) significant reductions in BP measured at the worksite as well as at the clinic where the training took place. In general, the worksite BPs were somewhat higher than clinic BPs: the worksite reductions in SBP were 67% of those measured in the clinic, while those for DBP were only 37%.

Agras, Taylor, Kraemer, Allen, and Schneider (1980) addressed this issue directly by measuring BP around the clock (every 15 minutes to 2 hours) on 5 hospitalized hypertensives who were given a brief but intensive course of relaxation training. Changes in BP immediately following the relaxation training ranged from 1 to 12 mm Hg. Moreover, it took on average about 60 minutes for BP to return to pretreatment levels after each relaxation session. Finally, there was statistically significant evidence of a generalized reduction in BP around the clock on the days relaxation training took place. This was most pronounced during sleep when SBP was about 12 mm Hg lower than on control days and DBP was about 8 mm Hg lower. These laboratory findings thus seem to confirm a generalized effect of relaxation on BP; moreover, they have important implications for the next topic, Home Practice.

Home Practice

As is obvious from the detailed instructions of our relaxation regimen, we place great emphasis on regular home practice of the various aspects of the relaxation program. Like many other investigators, we ask patients to practice at least once per day for 20 minutes. We also strongly suggest that two practices per day is better. The data on duration of relaxation effects on BP from the Agras et al. (1980) study support multiple practices per day at least in the very early stages (first 2 weeks) of treatment.

To check on reported home practice, we ask patients to keep a simple diary in which they record: (a) time of day of the home practice; (b) length of the practice; and (c) self-rating of relaxation on a 0 (not relaxed) to 10 (extremely relaxed) scale.

An elegant study of adherence to home practice was reported by the Agras group (Taylor, Agras, Schneider, & Allen, 1983). Patients were loaned tape recorders and a home-practice tape. The recorder contained a microprocessor circuit that recorded actual times the relaxation tape was played. Over the course of an 8-week relaxation-training regimen, Taylor et al. (1983) found patients actually practiced 4.6 times per week as opposed to a self-reported frequency of 5.9 times per week. Only 39% of the 23 patients were adhering strictly to the schedule. Interestingly, practice decreased from about 6 times per week for the first 2 weeks to about 2.5 times per week for the last 2 weeks.

Two other points emerged. First, the correlation between computer-recorded practice and self-reported practice was high:

r (21) = 0.88, p < .0001, indicating that one can have relative confidence in self-report of practice. Second, the correlations between frequency of practice, measured either way, and decrease in either SBP or DBP were all nonsignificant (and essentially zero). It could be that home practice is completely irrelevant. More likely is that home practice above some minimal level does not yield additional benefits. Regardless of this, we advise stressing regular home practice to patients.

Home practice after treatment is complete. One reason for stressing home practice during active treatment is to help the patient develop the habit of achieving a deeply relaxed state regularly so that the habit will persist. However, a clinical "fact of life" is that patients practice less frequently after formal treatment has ended. In fact, as noted in the Taylor et al. (1983) study, patients begin tapering off even during active treatment.

One possible way to maintain regular practice is through periodic booster sessions. In our own clinic (Blanchard et al., 1986) we found once-per-month booster-treatment sessions showed a trend (p = .24) toward having a *deleterious* effect. In a study of retraining initially successful patients who relapsed (BP rose toward baseline levels) Agras, Schneider, and Taylor (1984) found *no* advantage for active retraining versus periodic contact.

In Figure 4–2 we illustrate the effects of discontinuation of regular practice. This patient, a 45-year-old male, showed good compliance with home practice during treatment, but then a gradual discontinuation. There was a good treatment response (BP = −24/−17), which also began to lessen as practice was discontinued.

Home-Practice Audiotape

As described earlier, we routinely give patients an audiotape to guide home practice from the very first session. This seems to be a common practice (Agras et al., 1983). This usually accepted practice was recently subjected to an experimental test (Hoelscher, Lichstein, Fischer, & Hegarty, 1987). They assigned 48 hypertensives to receive either (a) PMR with a home practice audiotape; (b) PMR without the tape; or (c) a BP monitoring control.

Results showed significant reductions in BP for both treated groups with no statistical difference between them. However, by the 2-month follow-up, the group with the tape had a 93% greater reduction (6.4 mm Hg) in SBP than the no-tape PMR group, but only an 8% greater reduction in DBP. Despite the Hoelscher et al. findings, we would advise giving patients a home-practice audiotape.

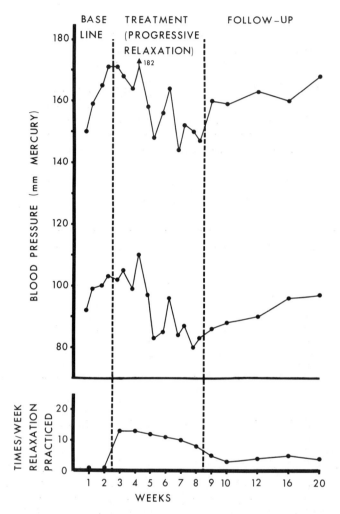

FIGURE 4–2. Effects on BP of Discontinuation of Practice

There are three primary values of the home-practice tape: (a) It controls the pace and duration of the home-practice session. On their own, many patients tend to rush through the exercises and report taking as little as 8 minutes to complete a session. With the tape, a full 20 to 25 minutes is used. We believe this is helpful. (b) Some patients report worrying about getting the sequence of exercises right. The tape eliminates this concern. While we do not believe there is anything magical or special about our sequence, relieving patients of this concern may help a few to become more relaxed.

Standard tape versus tailor-made tape. An issue you may want to consider is whether to give all patients a standard home-practice tape or whether a tape tailored for each specific patient should be used. In our work we have tried both ways and find no systematic advantage for one method over the other. We have had a few patients, who, after receiving a standard tape comment that they were surprised when the voice on the tape was not their therapist's voice.

We would advocate tailoring the tape to the patient for the following reasons: (a) it will be your voice instructing the patient; (b) if you include some relaxing imagery, it can be idiosyncratic to the patient; (c) if there are deviations from the standard procedure, such as omitting a muscle group or not using a particular filler suggestion, these can be incorporated.

Figure 4–3 consists of a complete transcript for a home-practice relaxation tape. It can give you an idea of pacing and pauses in the relaxation induction.

This is the tape for Week 1 of your relaxation training. You should be in a comfortable relaxed position, either sitting in a comfortable chair or lying in your bed. Be sure to loosen any tight or restrictive clothing. Now close your eyes and let yourself begin to relax. I will be giving you instructions to relax—just like the ones we went through on your first visit. Now I want you to tense your muscles in your right lower arm . . . study the tensions located in your arm . . . study those tensions . . . and now relax the muscles of your right lower arm . . . and study the difference between the tension and the relaxation. . . . Now I want you to tense the muscles in your left lower arm . . . study the tensions located in your left lower arm . . . study those tensions . . . and now relax the muscles of your left lower arm . . . and study the difference between the tension and the relaxation. . . . Now I want you to tense both of your lower arms together . . . tense both of your lower arms . . . focus on the tensions in your lower arms . . . study the tensions . . . and now relax the muscles of your lower arms and study the difference between the tension and the relaxation.

Just let yourself become more and more relaxed . . . if you feel yourself becoming drowsy that will be fine, too. If you think of relaxation and of letting go of your muscles . . . they will become more loose . . . heavy . . . and relaxed. . . . Just let your muscles go . . . as you become more deeply relaxed.

Now I want you to tense the muscles of your right, upper arm . . . study the tensions located in your right, upper arm . . . concentrate on those tensions . . . and now relax the muscles of your right, upper arm . . . and study the differences between the tension and the relaxation. . . . Now I want you to tense the muscles of your left, upper arm . . . study the tensions located in your left, upper arm . . . focus on those tensions . . . and relax the muscles of your left, upper arm . . . and study the difference between the tension and the relaxation. . . . Now I'd like you to tense the muscles of both of your upper arms together . . . study the tensions located in your upper arms . . . and study the difference between the tension and the relaxation . . . study the difference as you continue to relax. . . .

Now I want you to tense the muscles of your right, lower leg . . . study the tensions located in your lower leg . . . focus on the tensions . . . now relax the muscles of your lower leg . . . and study the difference between the tension and the relaxation. . . . Now I want you to tense the muscles of your left, lower leg . . . study the tensions located in your left, lower leg . . . study those tensions . . . now relax the muscles of your left, lower leg . . . and study the difference . . . between the tension and the relaxation. . . . Now I want you to tense both of your lower legs together . . . study the tensions located in your lower legs . . . study those tensions . . . now relax the muscles of your lower legs . . . and study the difference . . . between the tension . . . and the relaxation. . . .

You're becoming more and more relaxed . . . sleepy . . . sleepy . . . more relaxed. . . . As you become more relaxed . . . you will feel yourself settling deeply into the chair. . . . All your muscles are becoming more and more comfortably relaxed . . . loose . . . heavy . . . and relaxed. . . .

Now I want you to tense the muscles of both thighs together . . . study the tensions located in your thighs . . . study those tensions . . . now relax the muscles of your thighs . . . and study the difference . . . between the tension . . . and the relaxation. . . . Now I'd like you to tense the muscles of your abdomen . . . study the tensions located in your abdomen . . . focus on those tensions . . . now relax the muscles of your abdomen . . . and study the difference . . . between the tension . . . and the relaxation. . . . Now I'd like you to tense the muscles of your chest . . . take a deep breath . . . study the tensions located in your chest . . . study those tensions . . . now relax the muscles of your chest . . . and study the difference . . . between the tension . . . and the relaxation. . . .

The relaxation is growing deeper . . . and still deeper . . . you are relaxed . . . drowsy and relaxed . . . your breathing is regular . . . and relaxed. . . . With each breath you take in . . . your relaxation increases . . . and each time you exhale . . . you spread the relaxation throughout your body. . . . Now I want you to tense the muscles of your shoulders . . . study the tensions located in your shoulders . . . study those tensions . . . now relax the muscles of your shoulders . . . and study the difference . . . between the tension and the relaxation. . . . Now I want you to tense the muscles of your neck . . . study the tensions located in your neck . . . concentrate on the tensions in your neck . . . now relax the muscles of your neck . . . and study the difference . . . between the tension . . . and the relaxation. . . .

Note the pleasant feelings of warmth and heaviness . . . that are coming into your body. . . . As your muscles relax completely . . . you will always be clearly aware of what you are doing . . . and what I am saying . . . as you become more deeply relaxed. . . . Now I want you to tense the muscles of your lips . . . study the tensions located in your lips . . . study those tensions . . . now relax the muscles of your lips . . . study the difference . . . between the tension . . . and the relaxation. . . . Now I want you to tense the muscles of your eyes . . . study the tensions located in your eyes . . . study those tensions . . . now relax the muscles of your eyes . . . and study the difference . . . between the tension . . . and the relaxation. . . . Now I want you to tense the muscles of your lower forehead . . . study the tensions located in your lower forehead . . . study those tensions . . . now relax the muscles of your lower forehead . . . and study the difference . . . between the tension . . . and the relaxation. . . .

Now the very deep state of relaxation is moving through all areas of your body . . . you are becoming more and more comfortably relaxed . . . drowsy . . . and relaxed. . . . You can feel the comfortable sensations of relaxation . . . as you go into deeper . . . and deeper state . . . of relaxation. . . . Now I want you to tense the muscles of your upper forehead . . . study the tensions located in your upper forehead . . . study those tensions . . . now relax the muscles of your upper forehead . . . and study the difference between the tension . . . and the relaxation. . . .

Now I want you to relax all the muscles of your body . . . just let them become more and more relaxed . . . I'm going to help you to achieve a deeper state of relaxation . . . by counting from one to five. As I count, you will feel yourself becoming more and more deeply relaxed . . . farther and farther down . . . into a deep . . . restful state . . . of relaxation. . . . One. . . . You are going to become more deeply relaxed. . . . Two. . . . Down . . . down . . . into a very deep . . . relaxed state. . . . Three. . . . Four. . . . More and more relaxed . . . Five. . . . Deeply relaxed. . . . Now I want you to remain in a very relaxed state . . . and I want you to begin to attend just to your breathing . . . breathe through your nose . . . notice the cool air as you breathe in . . . and the warm, moist air . . . as you exhale. . . . Use your stomach muscles as you breathe . . . just continue to attend to your breathing . . . now each time you exhale . . . mentally repeat the words. . . . Relax. . . . Inhale. . . . Exhale. . . . Relax. . . . Inhale. . . . Exhale. . . . Relax . . . .
. . . .

Continue to concentrate on your breathing, but now try to imagine as clearly and as vividly as you can . . . that you are lying on a blanket . . . on a beautiful beach . . . in the summertime . . . the sky is a darkening, rich blue . . . and the burnt orange sun . . . is beginning to set over the ocean . . . you are watching the waves as they roll onto the shore . . . and roll back out again . . . in the distance . . . you can hear the cry of the sea birds . . . and the sound of the waves . . . as they roll onto the shore . . . and roll back out again. . . . The pleasant saltiness of the sea is in the air . . . you are enveloped by the warmth of the sun from above . . . and the warmth of the sand beneath the blanket. . . . Let the warmth pour into every muscle of your body . . . you are feeling very, very warm . . . and very, very relaxed . . . there is a cool breeze . . . and there is nothing for you to do . . . but concentrate on the great feelings of warmth . . . of pleasant relaxation . . . just flowing through every muscle of your body. . . . Just watch and listen to the waves . . . as they roll in and roll out again . . . you feel very pleasant and relaxed. . . . .
. . . .

Now I'm going to help you to return to your normal state of alertness. . . . In a little while . . . I will begin counting backwards from five to one . . . you will gradually become more alert. . . . When I reach two . . . I want you to open your eyes. . . . When I get to one . . . you will be entirely roused up . . . in your normal state of alertness. . . . Ready now. . . . Five. . . . Four. . . . You're becoming more and more alert . . . you feel very refreshed. . . . Three. . . . Two. . . . Now your eyes are open, you feel very alert and refreshed. . . . One. This is the end of the tape.

FIGURE 4–3. Transcript for Home-Practice Relaxation Tape

Weaning the patient from the audiotape. Although the major long-term goal of relaxation training for the hypertensive patient is reduction of BP, a primary intermediate goal is for the patient to be able to rapidly achieve a fairly deep relaxed state. Our whole relaxation regimen is aimed at this goal.

However, we have found that some patients become dependent upon the home-practice audiotape. We suggest that the patient stop using the audiotape on a daily basis during the second 4 weeks of training and, instead, begin to use it only every other day. On alternate days the patient should be practicing relaxation-by-recall. This schedule of tape-assisted relaxation can be thinned to once per 3 days and so on. It is, however, probably beneficial for the patient to go through the full 16-muscle-group sequence at home once or twice per week throughout treatment.

Gauging the Depth of Relaxation

A potential problem in relaxation training is knowing whether it has worked or not. Of course, one can rely on the ultimate clinical endpoint of BP reduction, but this is not very satisfactory in the short run and also operates on a logical fallacy. At the crudest level, one can ask the patient after the relaxation induction whether or not the patient was relaxed. This all-or-none scaling is not very precise.

A somewhat more sophisticated form of self-report, which we routinely used in our work, is to ask patients to gauge how relaxed they were using a 1-to-10 scale where 1 is *not relaxed* and 10 is *extremely relaxed*. Patients readily understand this approach, and it yields useful data. A problem, however, with the self-report rating of relaxation, common to all self-reports, is that of bias. Patients will sometimes report what they believe the therapist wants to hear.

Schilling and Poppen (1983) devised a less reactive method of gauging depth of relaxation, their Behavioral Relaxation Rating Scale. In this scale, 10 different behaviors are scored over a 60-second observation interval.

This scale is described more fully in Table 4–4.

Schilling and Poppen have presented reliability and validity data on their scale. Our own use of it tends to confirm their validity reports.

Table 4-4. *BEHAVIORAL RELAXATION SCALE*
Don Schilling and Roger Poppen
Rehabilitation Institute
Southern Illinois University
Carbondale, Illinois 62901

1. *Breathing**
Unrelaxed: (1) Equal or higher frequency than baseline. (2) Irregularities that disrupt the rhythm of breathing such as coughing, laughing, sneezing, sniffing, swallowing, yawning, hiccupping, or vocalizations (excluding nasal sounds resulting from loud breathing). (3) Movement that prevents frequency observation.
Relaxed: Lower frequency than baseline with none of the above irregularities observed.

2. *Quiet*
Unrelaxed: Any vocalizations (not necessarily a verbalization). This includes talking, sighs, grunts, or nasal sounds (e.g., loud exhale through nose).
Relaxed: No vocalizations or nasal sounds.

3. *Body*
Unrelaxed: (1) Any movement of chest, waist, or hip area except for respiration (e.g., shifting position in the chair). (2) Any movement of arms or legs that does *not* cause movement of head, shoulders, hands, or feet (these are scored separately). (3) Any part of back or hips lifted from reclined position.
Relaxed: No movement of chest, waist, hips, arms, or legs. Body resting against chair.

4. *Head*
Unrelaxed: (1) Head unsupported by recliner. (2) Head deviating from body midline. The entire structure of the nose must be beyond the midline. In most cases the midline can be discriminated by buttons or other clothing features (e.g., the apex of a V neck) that bisect the body longitudinally. (3) Head tilted upward or downward or to one side. (4) Movement of head.
Relaxed: Head supported by the recliner and in the midline of body (i.e., any part of the nose transected by midline).

5. *Eyes*
Unrelaxed: (1) Eyes open. (2) Eyelids closed but wrinkled or fluttering. (3) Eye movement beneath eyelids.
Relaxed: Closed with eyelids showing a smooth appearance.

Table 4-4. *Continued*

6. *Mouth*

   Unrelaxed: (1) Lips closed at center of mouth. (2) Mouth open beyond approximately 1 inch at center. In most cases the corners of the mouth will separate when lips part beyond criterion at center, for example when smiling. (3) Clenched teeth is also considered evidence of an unrelaxed mouth. This criterion should not be used, though, if dental structure prevents discrimination. (4) Talking. (5) Tongue movement (e.g., licking lips).

   Relaxed: Lips slightly parted at center of mouth (approximately $\frac{1}{4}"$–$1"$, or about the width of one's index finger) with teeth unclenched if the latter is discriminable (see above).

7. *Throat* (see neck)

   Unrelaxed: (1) Noticeable movement in the throat (e.g., swallowing, larynx moving). (2) Twitches in neck muscles.

   Relaxed: No swallowing or other movements.

8. *Shoulders*

   Unrelaxed: (1) Shoulders on a diagonal plane. (2) Both shoulders transect same horizontal plane but are raised or lowered so as not to appear rounded. (3) Movement of shoulders. (4) Shoulders raised from chair.

   Relaxed: Both shoulders appear rounded and transect the same horizontal plane; no movement; resting against chair.

9. *Hands*

   Unrelaxed: (1) Hands clenching armrest. (2) Fingers intertwined. (3) Fingers extended so as to appear straight or render the back of hand concave. (4) Fingers excessively curled to the extent that the nails are exposed to the same surface to which the palms are facing. (A fist is the most obvious example of the latter.) (5) Fingers extending over side of armrest.

   Relaxed: Hand appears clawlike. That is, hanging with palms down and fingers slightly curled. All fingers of both hands must be curled but are not required to remain on armrest. Fingers (excluding thumb) are considered "slightly" curled if a standard pencil can pass freely beneath at the highest point of the arc.

10. *Feet*

    Unrelaxed: (1) Feet pointing vertically or at an angle less than 30° with respect to each other. (2) Feet pointing away from each other at angle greater than 90°. (3) Feet crossed. (4) Movement of feet. (5) Heels more than one inch in front or behind each other.

    Relaxed: Pointed away from each other at approximately 60° to 90° angle, i.e., the angle between the midline of foot and the footrest in between 30° and 60°.

Procedure

1-minute observation/record intervals:

   30 sec — observe frequency of breaths
   15 sec — observe behaviors 2–10 concurrently
   15 sec — record breathing frequency and score observations of items 2–10.

Notes: 1. Behaviors 2–10 scoring not to be noted during breathing-interval observations.
       2. Scoring includes behaviors occurring in interval cues.

(Reproduced with the permission of Dr. Roger Poppen, Table 7-5)

*One breath equals one inhale-exhale cycle. Included are any part of an inhale occurring on the cue signalling the end of the observation period.

Thus, use of this rating scale by the trainer at the end of a relaxation induction should provide a valid check on patient self-report of relaxation.

Discrepancies of either sort (patient claiming to be deeply relaxed while observation does not confirm, or observations showing deep relaxation that the patient denies) are bothersome. If the patient denies relaxation, it may be because of a worry or cognitive-activity component. This should be explored and if this is the case, more emphasis should be put on breath counting and calming mental imagery.

Comments on the Relaxation Training Regimen

The best setting for conducting relaxation training, in our opinion, is a quiet, relatively sound-attenuated room in which the lighting can be dimmed.

All of our treatment has been done with the patient sitting in a high-backed recliner with the footrest up to support the legs. Although a recliner is not necessary, a comfortable chair is important. We also believe the chair should have a back high enough to support the neck and head easily.

The trainer should, of course, use a calm, soothing voice tone. We believe that conducting the relaxation training live, rather than by audiotape, is important. Almost every *treatment* study using PMR has conducted the relaxation live. There is some research (Paul & Trimble, 1970) that gives empirical support to this view. Furthermore, when conducting it live, the clinician can spot problems, such as the patients not tensing a muscle group properly, and correct it. Finally, we suspect that the trainer makes small adjustments to the protocol based on feedback received, even nonverbally, from the patient.

We should make the following observations about our relaxation-training regimen:

1. There is nothing magical about the muscle-group sequence. Another sequence, more to the liking of a particular therapist, could be used.
2. There is nothing magical about the filler suggestions. Other phrasing that incorporates the same ideas could be used.

Despite these disclaimers, we remind the reader that it is the regimen described here that we have used and for which evaluative data are available in this book and in our various journal publications.

Thus, a therapist might want to omit some of the sessions to shorten the duration of the treatment. Many other investigators have used fewer sessions and shorter lengths of training with good results (e.g., Taylor et al., 1977).

Potential problems. There are three potential problems one may run into with this relaxation-training regimen. First, the relaxation induction is similar to one form of hypnotic induction, especially with the use of frequent suggestions. If patients have had experience with hypnosis, they may recognize this similarity and ask questions about it. Our standard reply is that the training is not hypnosis, but it is similar in certain ways. Along these lines it is important to use between-exercise suggestion 7 (see pp. 53), which explicitly tells the patient that "he is clearly aware of what he is doing."

A second problem is that of so-called relaxation-induced anxiety. Heide and Borkovec (1983) have discussed this problem and documented its occurrence. We have not had this problem in our 50 hypertensive patients treated with abbreviated PMR. We have seen this problem occasionally (about one instance in 150 patients or 1200 to 1500 sessions) in our work with chronic headache (Blanchard & Andrasik, 1985). These reactions range from a sudden, but mild, increase in anxiety all the way to a full-blown panic attack. Should this occur, we suggest the following: (a) It is important that the therapist remain calm. (b) Reassure the patient that everything is all right. Have him sit up for a few minutes and even walk around the room if necessary. (c) Then resume the relaxation training.

It is important that the aversive thoughts and sensations that accompany the panic attack not be conditioned to the consulting room, to the therapist, or to the treatment situation in general. The preceding steps should help prevent that.

A third problem is muscle spasms. These seem more frequent in males than females and probably result from the patient's tensing the particular muscle group too intensely. A painful muscle spasm certainly will disrupt the overall state of relaxation. To handle this problem: (a) stop the relaxation indication and have the patient try to relax or massage the affected muscle group until the spasm has decreased, and (b) then resume the relaxation training after warning the patient not to tense muscles so hard. Avoid the spasmed group as you continue the induction.

RELAXATION RESPONSE

The *Relaxation Response* (RR) is a term coined by Herbert Benson (1975) for his secularized version of Transcendental Meditation (TM). The essence of this relaxation technique is the regular practice of mantra meditation, a very passive form of relaxation. Although mantra meditation has a very long history (Benson, 1975), it is only in the last 10 to 15 years that it has been subjected to systematic scientific study as a possible nondrug treatment for essential hypertension.

Benson and his colleagues published several uncontrolled studies of the use of RR (partly as TM, partly as PR) with essential hypertensives. They are summarized in Table 4–5. Since then there have been a number of controlled studies that have used the RR. The essential results of several of these are presented in Table 4–6.

Table 4-5. Uncontrolled Studies of the Relaxation Response with Hypertension

Authors	No. of subjects	Length of training (weeks)	Pretreatment BP	Posttreatment BP	Change in BP
Benson et al. (1973)	30	9	150/93	135/not given	15/——
Benson et al. (1974b)	14	20	146/92	135/87	11/5
Benson et al. (1974a)	22	25	147/95	140/91	7/4
Blackwell et al. (1976)	7	12	135/98	131/96	4/2
Pollack et al. (1977)	20	26	155/96	149/94	6/2

Examining the results in Tables 4–5 and 4–6, one can see that Benson and his colleagues consistently achieved statistically significant, but sometimes fairly small, decreases in BP across the 3 studies. The replication attempts by Blackwell et al. (1976) and Pollack et al. (1977) yielded only minimal decreases in SBP and DBP.

The picture that emerges from the controlled studies is more mixed. While Stone and DeLeo (1976) showed a substantial reduction in BP that was significantly greater than found in the control condition, other tests of the procedure are not as promising, especially the repeated efforts of Dave Shapiro and his colleagues. An especially interesting comparison is in the study by Goldstein et al. (1982), which compared RR to routine antihypertensive drug therapy. The drugs were clinically and statistically superior.

Table 4-6. Controlled Evaluations of Relaxation Response (RR) with Hypertension

Authors	No. of Ss	Control condition	Length of training	Pretreatment BP	Posttreatment BP	Change BP
Stone & DeLeo (1976)	19	C (n = 5) monthly BP measurement	6 months	RR 146/95	131/85	15/10
				C 148/93	145/93	3/0
Goldstein, Shapiro et al. (1982)	24	D drugs, mainly diuretics	3 months	RR 150/97	151/101	-1/-4
		C Home monitoring of BP		D 144/98	141/99	14/6
				C 141/96	141/99	0/-3
Seer & Raeburn (1980)	27	C Pretesting & Posttesting only	13 weeks	RR 152/104	148/97	4/7
				C 150/102	152/104	-2/-2
Surwit, Shapiro, & Good (1978)	16	C EMG Biofeedback	10 weeks	RR 141/NA	136/NA	4/—
				C 136/NA	133/NA	3/—

Results with RR by the Present Authors

In the small-scale comparison of various relaxation techniques described earlier (Blanchard et al., 1979) eight similar patients received 12 individually administered sessions of RR over a 6-week period. Regular home practice was expected and monitored. The BP values for these 8 patients at baseline, end-of-treatment, and at a 3-month follow-up are given in Table 4–7.

Table 4-7. BP Results from Training in Relaxation Response

	Baseline	1-Week Posttreatment	3-Month Posttreatment
SBP	151.4	141.6	155.6
DBP	95.8	90.4	94.6

As one can see from Table 4–7, the initial response to treatment was fairly good with a 10 mm Hg decrease in SBP and 5 mm decrease in DBP. However, by 3 months posttreatment, the treatment effects were gone in DBP and SBP was 4 mm Hg *higher* than baseline.

As best we could determine, regularity of practice of the RR failed during follow-up. Benson et al. (1974) have noted a similar relapse in BP when patients fail to meditate or practice on a regular basis.

Protocol for Teaching Relaxation Response

The RR is by far the simplest relaxation technique to teach. Instruction and initial practice take only a few minutes. The Instructions we have used were taken from Benson's (1975) book:

1. Select a quiet place where you are unlikely to be disturbed for 10 to 20 minutes.
2. Select a comfortable chair. Although it does not need to be a recliner with head and neck support, use of such a chair is a good idea. A sitting position is preferable to a bed because one does not want to fall asleep.
3. Allow yourself to become comfortably relaxed all over.
4. Breathe through your nose and attend to your breathing.
5. Each time as you exhale, mentally repeat the word *One* to yourself.
6. If you find thoughts coming into mind, very gently push them aside and return to mentally repeating the word *One* with each exhalation.

Comments on RR. A sizeable proportion of patients does not seem to like the RR procedure. This may be because of its simplicity; we suspect the more involved ritual of PMR holds patients to the regular practice regimen better.

Some patients do not seem able to sustain the relaxed, meditative state. Intrusive thoughts and worries are such that they are not able to continue the meditation. It is probably the case that this type of individual is most in need of the mental calm of meditation and would benefit from it a great deal.

This form of relaxation lends itself readily to transfer to the workplace. Peters, Benson, and Peters (1977) conducted a major controlled trial at the worksite. Office workers were assigned to either (a) RR, (b) sitting quietly for comparable periods to the RR group, or (c) BP measurement only. Workers took two 15-minute relaxation breaks daily during the work week. As a whole, the sample was not hypertensive (117/76). Those who practiced RR for 12 weeks had decreases in BP of 6.7/5.2 millimeters of mercury, which was significantly greater than that found for those who merely rested (2.6/2.0) or did not rest (0.5/1.2). Those subjects from the RR condition ($n = 20$) who were borderline hypertensive (137/90) showed the greatest decrease in BP (12.2/8.4). There was good acceptance of the program, at least in the short term.

Summary. RR is by far the simplest relaxation technique to teach to patients. Treatment response has been highly variable, with the bulk of recent studies not finding very impressive results. Moreover, in our experience, long-term compliance is fairly poor.

AUTOGENIC TRAINING

Autogenic training (to be abbreviated AT hereafter) was developed in Germany by Johannes Schultz and popularized in this country by Wolfgang Luthe (1977). In its simplest form AT seems to be a combination of passive-relaxation exercises combined with meditation and specific self-instruction. The form of AT most widely used in this country evolved from the work of Luthe (1977) and focuses on six so-called standard autogenic formula.

Pikoff (1984) recently published a review of all of the studies which used AT in the USA as of 1984. There were only 30 studies. Very few of them used AT alone as a treatment condition. Instead, a brief version of AT utilizing only two of the standard exercises has frequently been combined with thermal biofeedback, especially in the treatment of migraine headache and Raynaud's disease.

As a result of a professional-exchange program with the USSR, sponsored by NHLBI, one of us (EBB) became familiar with work by various Soviet investigators on the use of AT with hypertension. All of this work appeared in Russian-language journals and much of it is uncontrolled. However, from the available translations AT did appear to be effective.

SUNY-AMC Hypertension Project

We are just completing the American half of a cross-cultural comparison (with scientists at the Cardiology Institute in Moscow) of AT with thermal biofeedback. The version of AT used in this study was developed by Dr. Boris Salenko, a Russian psychiatrist. Our data on AT comes exclusively from this study and is based on the treatment of 13 unmedicated patients (12 male/1 female, average age 44) with mild hypertension. In this study patients were seen for 20 outpatient visits at the rate of approximately twice per week. The results are presented in Table 4–8.

As can be seen, we had a 5-millimeter reduction in SBP and a 7-millimeter = mercury reduction in DBP, which was both statistically and clinically significant ($p = .005$).

Table 4-8. Authors' BP Results from Autogenic Training

	Pretreatment	Posttreatment	t	p
SBP	139.9	134.9	1.47	0.17
DBP	96.8	89.4	3.55	0.005
$N = 13$				

Autogenic Training Protocol

As noted above, the AT protocol used called for 20 outpatient sessions on a twice-per-week basis. This seemed somewhat excessive and could probably be shortened to 12 to 16 sessions. The same kind of setting was used as with PMR: a sound-attenuated room in which the illumination level could be reduced somewhat. Patients sat in recliners with both their legs supported and their head and neck supported.

A key feature of this particular version of AT was the Relaxation Figure, a somewhat complex geometric figure done in shades of black and gray. The patient is instructed to focus upon the figure while repeating the autogenic phrases and bringing on the sensations of relaxation. It appears to be a very Pavlovian model of training in which the sensations of relaxation are repeatedly paired with the Figure so that, later, mentally recalling the Figure will lead to the sensations of relaxation.

Sessions are introduced with a brief passage of music (about 90 seconds) and end with music also.

The phrases are spoken by the trainer in a clear, authoritative voice. The patient is instructed to repeat the phrase to himself and as he repeats it, to try to experience the feelings and sensations he has described. All of the phrases are couched in first person. Thus, a key feature is to allow enough time between phrases for the patient to repeat the instruction to himself and then to focus his attention on his body so as to experience the feeling. (One way for the *trainer* to control the timing is to mentally repeat the phrase to himself and then scan the body part during the silent interval.)

Rationale for Patients. The AT is introduced with the following:

We are going to begin your relaxation training today. You will be learning something known as Autogenic Training. It is a passive, meditative form of relaxation and self-instruction. This procedure has been used extensively in Russia and found to be a very successful treatment for hypertension. We are testing it in this country. The idea behind Autogenic Training is that regular practice of relaxation—especially this form of relaxation, which focuses in part on the autonomic or involuntary part of the nervous system—and incorporation of this relaxation into your everyday life, will lead to a reduction in overall level of arousal and subsequently to a reduction in blood pressure.

Verbatim Autogenic Training Protocol for First Session

Initial Instructions:
a. Make yourself comfortable.
b. Concentrate on feelings of relaxation, peace and calmness.
c. Repeat to yourself mentally the phrases I say and then try to feel and experience the sensations or feelings described in your own body.
d. Be very attentive to my voice and to the sensations and feelings in your body.
   1. I am becoming calm. . . .
      I am becoming calmer and calmer. . . .
      My attention is focused inward. . . .
      Nothing distracts me, nothing keeps me from concentrating my attention on the sensations in my body. . . .

2. I am calm . . . absolutely calm.
   My breathing is calm, deep and regular.
   My head is clear and light.
   My attention is focused on the relaxation formulas.
   I am absolutely calm.
3. I feel the pleasant warmth sweeping over my body. . . .
   The warmth brings relaxation. . . .
   The warmth brings lightness . . . pleasant lightness . . . and comfortable relaxation. . . .
   I am absolutely calm . . . and relaxed. . . .
4. I am calm . . . absolutely calm. . . .
   I am concentrating on the relaxation formulas. . . .
   I feel pleasant warmth enveloping my feet. . . .
   My feet are warm . . . relaxed . . . comfortably relaxed . . . comfortably warm. . . .
5. I am absolutely calm. . . .
   My feet are relaxed, comfortable and warm . . . comfortably relaxed. . . .
   I feel the pleasant warmth go up my legs. . . .
   My calf muscles are becoming warm and relaxed. . . .
   The warmth is enveloping my knees. . . .
   The warmth goes up my thighs. . . .
   My legs feel relaxed, comfortable and warm. . . .
   Comfortably relaxed . . . comfortably warm. . . .
6. I am absolutely calm. . . .
   I feel warmth throughout my whole body all the way up to my abdomen. . . .
   My abdomen is relaxed, comfortable and warm. . . .
   The warmth envelopes my buttocks. . . .
   My waist becomes warmer. . . .
   The warmth goes up the spine. . . .
   It reaches the back of my neck and head. . . .
   My back feels warm . . . relaxed. . . .
   My back and shoulders are relaxed, comfortable and warm. . . .
   comfortably relaxed . . . comfortably warm. . . .
   My neck muscles are deeply relaxed. . . .
   My muscles in the back of my head feel very comfortably relaxed. . . .
   My neck and head are relaxed, comfortable and warm. . . .
   All of my body is warm and relaxed . . . warm and pleasantly relaxed. . . .
7. I am absolutely calm. . . .
   My body is warm and relaxed. . . .
   I feel pleasant warmth envelop my hands. . . .

My hands are becoming warm . . . and relaxed. . . .
Comfortably relaxed . . . comfortably warm. . . .
I can feel the warm blood pulsing in my fingers. . . .
My hands are relaxed, comfortable and warm. . . .
I am absolutely calm. . . .

8. My hands are warm and relaxed. . . .
The warmth envelopes my lower arms. . . .
The warmth moves to my upper arms. . . .
The warmth now envelopes my whole arms. . . .
My arms are warm and relaxed, pleasantly warm and relaxed. . . .
I am absolutely calm. . . .

9. My hands are warm and relaxed. . . .
My fingers are warm and relaxed. . . .
My palms are warm. . . .
My wrists are warm. . . .
My forearms are warm. . . .
My whole arms are warm and relaxed, pleasantly warm and relaxed. . . .
I am absolutely calm. . . .

10. My mouth muscles are becoming more . . . and still more, deeply relaxed. . . .
My forehand muscles are becoming relaxed. . . .
My eye muscles are becoming relaxed. . . .
My eyelids feel very relaxed. . . .
My lips are becoming relaxed. . . .
My tongue is becoming relaxed. . . .
It rests at the bottom of my mouth . . . limp . . . relaxed. . . .
My whole face is warm, comfortable, and relaxed . . . comfortably relaxed. . . .
I am absolutely calm. . . .

11. My whole body feels warm . . . relaxed . . . loose. . . .
Pleasantly loose . . . comfortably relaxed . . . comfortably warm. . . .
I haven't the slightest wish to stir. . . .
My legs are loose . . . and relaxed. . . .
My arms are loose . . . and relaxed. . . .
My back is relaxed. . . .
The muscles in the back of my neck and head feel relaxed. . . .
My facial muscles are relaxed. . . .
My breathing is regular, calm, deep, and relaxed. . . .
My head is clear. . . .
My forehead feels pleasantly cool. . . .
My weariness or fatigue leaves me . . . my worries and troubles leave me. . . .

12. I am absolutely calm. . . .

Nothing prevents me from concentrating on the relaxation formulas. . . .

My attention is turned inward. . . .

My mind is blank. . . .

I am absolutely calm. . . .

13. The feelings of relaxation are growing deeper and still deeper. . . .

My legs are deeply relaxed . . . and loose. . . .

My arms feel loose . . . and relaxed. . . .

My back is relaxed . . . I feel myself sinking into the chair. . . .

17. And *Now*

I feel joy, cheerfulness, energy, and strength spread throughout my body. . . .

My body becomes alert, and energetic. . . .

The waves of strength, power, energy are moving through all the areas of my body. . . .

I am strong . . . ready to act . . . powerful. . . .

My will is becoming strong . . . stronger and stronger. . . .

I am master of my body. . . .

18. And now I begin counting from 1 to 3 . . . then I will take a deep breath and open my eyes. . . .

So. . . . One. . . . Two. . . . Three. . . .

I've had a good rest, my whole body feels very refreshed.

Final Instructions

Have everyone take a deep breath and stretch.

Note: At later sessions the content of Item 13 changes and Items 14, 15 and 16 are added as noted below.

Changes in AT Protocol for Later Sessions

For Session 3, Item 13 is changed as outlined below and Items 14 and 15 are added:

13. The feelings of relaxation are growing deeper and still deeper. . . .

My legs are deeply relaxed . . . and loose. . . .

My arms feel loose . . . and relaxed. . . .

My back is relaxed . . . I feel myself sinking into the chair. . . .

The position of my body makes no difference to me. . . .

The position of my arms makes no difference to me. . . .

The position of my legs makes no difference to me. . . .

The position of my head makes no difference to me. . . .

I am absolutely calm. . . .

14. My body feels like it is melting and dissolving. . . .

I stop attending to my body. . . .

I stop feeling my body. . . .
My body is light. . . .
The position of my body makes no difference to me. . . .
I keep remembering this state of lightness, state of weightlessness and floating on air. . . .
Resting, floating, soaring, lightness. . . .
I am at peace with myself. . . .
I feel completely calm. . . .
I am absolutely calm. . . .

15. I am again trying to remember this state. . . .
    The state of lightness, weightlessness and floating on air. . . .
    My feelings and emotions are in full harmony. . . .
    I am at peace with myself. . . .
    I am absolutely calm. . . .

16. I like this state of peaceful calm, and relaxation . . . of floating and lightness. . . .
    I can reproduce this state at will, at any time, in any situation. . . .
    In any situation, at any time, I can reproduce this state of relaxation, of calm, of floating on air, of soaring as I am doing now. . . .
    And now I am once more absorbing, once more remembering the lightness and the floating. . . .
    The pleasant lightness of this state. . . .
    I am at peace and my mind and body in harmony. . . .

For Sessions 4 and 5, Item 13 is again changed to read:

13. The feelings of relaxation are growing deeper and still deeper. . . .
    My legs are deeply relaxed . . . and loose. . . .
    My arms feel loose . . . and relaxed. . . .
    My back is relaxed . . . I feel myself sinking into the chair. . . .
    My whole body feels light. . . .
    My arms are light. . . .
    My legs are light. . . .
    My breathing is calm . . . regular . . . deep . . . and relaxed. . . .
    My head is clear. . . .
    I feel light and serene. . . .

The protocol changes slightly for Items 14, 15, 16 beginning in Session 6. This same protocol is used for Sessions 6 through 20.

14. My body feels like it it is melting and dissolving. . . .
    I stop attending to my body. . . .
    I stop feeling my body. . . .
    My body is light. . . .
    The position of my body makes no difference to me. . . .

I keep remembering this state of lightness, state of weightlessness
and floating on air. . . .
Resting, floating, soaring, lightness. . . .
I am at peace with myself. . . .
I feel completely calm, peaceful and relaxed. . . .
I am absolutely calm. . . .
I imagine the relaxation figure. . . .
The figure makes me calm and relaxed. . . .
The figure helps me to remember and recreate this state. . . .
15. I am again trying to remember this state. . . .
The state of lightness, weightlessness and floating on air. . . .
The figure helps me to remember and recreate this state. . . .
My feelings and emotions are in full harmony. . . .
I am at peace with myself. . . .
I am at peace with sensations and feelings. . . .
I am absolutely calm. . . .
16. I like this state of peaceful calm, and relaxation . . . of floating and
lightness. . . .
The figure will help me reproduce this state. . . .
I can reproduce this state at will, at any time, in any situation. . . .
In any situation, at any time, I can reproduce this state of relaxation,
of calm, of floating on air, or soaring as I am doing now. . . .
And now I am once more absorbing, once more remembering the
lightness and the floating. . . .
The pleasant lightness of this state. . . .
I am at peace and my mind and body in harmony. . . .

Clinical Notes and Comments

It is obvious that there is a very Pavlovian-conditioning flavor to this
form of AT: One is repeatedly pairing the physical experience of
relaxation with the conditioned stimulus of the relaxation figure in the
expectation that memory, or a mental image, of the figure will bring on
automatically a sense of relaxation. For patients with any background in
psychology, this aspect of the training is obvious. We have readily
admitted it as if it were a positive feature.

Between 10% and 20% of a very small sample of patients did not like
the AT at all and dropped out. One patient seemed to have a great deal
of difficulty with "control" issues and, each time he was becoming very
relaxed, he would suddenly become very aroused. This is reminiscent of
Heide & Borkovec's (1983) "relaxation-induced anxiety."

The trainer has to work at not rushing through the protocol but
instead allowing the patient enough time to repeat the phrase to himself
and then try to generate the experience.

Home practice. As with the other relaxation procedures described in this chapter, regular home practice is important. We routinely gave the patients a tape of the Session 4 protocol to use at home. We asked for one 20-to-25-minute practice per day plus two brief 5-minute practices, one after arising in the morning and another in the evening.

REGULAR RELAXATION
PRACTICE

We conclude this section on relaxation techniques with some additional observations from one of our laboratories (EBB). In several studies (Blanchard, Miller, et al., 1979; Blanchard, Murphy, et al., 1979) we have used as a control condition having patients relax regularly on their own. The instructions and procedures have been very simple: The patients have come to the laboratory twice per week for about 30 minutes. During that time they are asked to relax on their own in a recliner located in a quiet, dimly lit room and then BP was taken. They have also been asked to relax on their own for about 20 minutes per day. No other formal instruction has been given.

The results with this procedure, across three studies, are summarized in Table 4–9.

Table 4-9. BP Results from Regular Self-Relaxation

Study	Sample size	Pretreatment BP	Posttreatment BP	Follow-up BP
Blanchard, Miller, et al. (1979)	10	149/88	141/83	143/85
Blanchard, Murphy, et al. (1979)	8	151/97	142/87	131/87
Blanchard et al. (1986)	4	135/94	134/93	——

As can be seen, this very simple control condition was moderately effective in one study (Blanchard, Murphy, et al., 1979) and very effective in another study (Blanchard, Miller, et al., 1979). In the latter study, it appeared that the excellent follow-up results were due in large part to faithful continuation of regular relaxation practice.

Chapter 5

Stress Management: Biofeedback Therapies

As mentioned in the Overview in Chapter 4, another major stress-management procedure that has been used extensively to treat hypertension includes several varieties of *biofeedback*, which has been defined as "a process in which a person learns to reliably influence physiological responses of two kinds: either responses which are not ordinarily under voluntary control or responses which ordinarily are easily regulated but for which regulation has broken down due to trauma or disease" (Blanchard & Epstein, 1978, p. 2).

The use of biofeedback as a treatment for hypertension is almost as old as the use of relaxation, dating to the early 1970s. We will discuss three forms of biofeedback that have been used to treat hypertension: (a) direct feedback of BP; (b) thermal biofeedback; and (c) frontal EMG biofeedback. The latter form of biofeedback is, in many ways, another form of relaxation training and could have been considered in that portion of Chapter 4.

DIRECT FEEDBACK OF BLOOD PRESSURE

Beginning in the late 1960s, David Shapiro, Bernard Tursky and their colleagues published a series of studies showing that, when subjects were given direct feedback of BP, they could reliably change it to a statistically significant degree (Shapiro, Tursky, Gershon, & Stern, 1969; Shapiro, Tursky, & Schwartz, 1970). Included in this initial work was a very important study (Benson, Shapiro, Tursky, & Schwartz, 1971) in which seven patients with essential hypertension were treated with the Direct BP Biofeedback procedure. Five of the seven showed large-scale (at least 16 mm Hg) decreases in SBP from a very stable baseline over treatment regimens ranging from 8 to 33 sessions.

The essence of the Direct BP Biofeedback procedure was the device that enabled the patient on a heartbeat-by-heartbeat basis to receive feedback of the relative value of SBP or DBP. For SBP (which has been the most frequently used) a BP cuff was inflated to above SBP and then gradually bled down until the first Korotkoff sound (see Chapter 3) could be detected. The patient's task was to make the Korotkoff sounds disappear by lowering SBP below the cuff pressure. A trial lasted 50 or 60 heartbeats and then the cuff was deflated to restore normal circulation for a few seconds. Next the cuff was reinflated to the previous level and the patient would again seek to lower SBP. After the patient was successful at one fixed cuff pressure, the pressure was automatically lowered by 2 mm Hg so as to continually challenge the patient on each succeeding trial. This so-called constant-cuff method was the subject of many experiments by Shapiro and his colleagues and continues to be used by them.

By the mid-1970s several other investigators, using similar technology, had published small-scale studies, usually uncontrolled, of the successful treatment of hypertension with Direct BP Biofeedback (Miller, 1972; Elder, Ruiz, Deabler, & Dillenkoffer, 1973; Kristt & Engel, 1975).

In our laboratory (Blanchard, Young, & Haynes, 1975) we developed a form of Direct BP Biofeedback that provided readings on a once-per-minute basis. The first four patients included in the report were successful in obtaining clinically meaningful decreases in SBP (average decrease 23.7 mm Hg).

Failure to replicate. After the initial round of successes, there next appeared a series of studies, usually with more patients and better controls, which failed to replicate the initial findings, again including one of our own (Blanchard, Miller, Abel, Haynes, & Wicker, 1979). In Table 5–1 is summarized this puzzling experience with Direct BP Biofeedback.

To the credit of Shapiro, he and his colleagues continued to study the constant-cuff method of Direct BP Biofeedback. In one other study (Surwit, Shapiro, & Good, 1978) it was not successful (ΔSBP = 0 mm Hg; $n = 8$). In an important later study (Goldstein, Shapiro, Thananopavarem, & Sambhi, 1982) it was relatively successful. In this study, Direct BP Biofeedback was compared to drug treatment and, to a monitoring of BP control over an 8-week period. As can be seen in Table

Table 5-1. Biofeedback and Hypertension: the Failure to Replicate

	Initial Report		Later Report	
Authors	Results	Authors	Results
Benson et al., 1971	$\Delta BP = -17$ mm 5/7 improved	Schwartz & Shapiro, 1973	$\Delta BP = 0$ 1/7 improved
Miller, 1972	$\Delta BP = 21$ mm one patient	Miller, 1975	Failure in 27 cases
Elder et al., 1973	$\Delta BP = -20\%$ of baseline	Elder & Eustis, 1975	$\Delta BP = -8$ mm 9/22 improved
Blanchard et al., 1975	$\Delta BP = 26$ mm 4/4 improved	Blanchard et al., 1979	$\Delta BP = 7$ mm

5–2, while drugs were much more effective on SBP than biofeedback, for DBP the two were essentially equivalent.

The Columbia Health Plan study. One other major study of the Direct BP Biofeedback procedure was conducted by Bernard Engel and his colleagues (Engel, Gaarder & Glasgow, 1981; Glasgow, Gaarder, & Engel, 1982; Engel, Glasgow, & Gaarder, 1983) on 127 patients. The bulk of the treatment—either a set of relaxation procedures or a direct BP biofeedback procedure—was self-administered by the patients at home on a regular (several times per day) basis.

The Direct BP Biofeedback consisted of teaching patients to take their own BP and then to use a variation of the constant-cuff procedure: The patient was trained to inflate the BP cuff to about SBP and to try to inhibit brachial artery sounds. Patients were instructed to attempt to control brachial artery sounds for about 25 to 30 seconds, after which

Table 5-2. Summary of Laboratory BPs from Goldstein et al. (1982)

	Baseline (no drugs)		End of treatment		Changes	
	SBP	DBP	SBP	DBP	SBP	DBP
Direct BP Biofeedback	149.1	97.3	145.0	92.9	−4.1	−4.4
Drugs	144.2	98.2	129.4	92.6	−14.8	−5.6
Self-monitoring ($n = 9$ per group)	141.2	96.2	144.7	98.8	+3.5	+2.6

they were to deflate the cuff for about 15 seconds. If successful in inhibiting 25% of sounds on the previous trial, the patient was told to inflate the cuff to a pressure level 2 mm Hg less than that on the previous trial. This procedure was repeated until the patient could no longer lower SBP on two consecutive trials (Glasgow et al., 1982, p. 158).

Patients who were given instruction in both biofeedback and relaxation tended to do better than those who practiced only one procedure or the other or who merely monitored BP. At a 6-month follow-up, one such two-treatment group had decreases of $-13.8/-10.2$ millimeters of mercury.

Conclusions

For the one of us (EBB) with experience with direct BP biofeedback, it has not been a satisfactory procedure primarily because of its lack of reliability. While some patients ($n = 2$) seem to have been helped a great deal by it in the controlled evaluation (Blanchard, Miller, et al., 1979), its lack of uniformity had led us personally to abandon it. The Engel procedure described above does, however, seem worth trying. On a clinical basis, combining this self-administered constant-cuff procedure with relaxation might prove very valuable for certain patients. It seems worth a try when other stress-management procedures are not working.

THERMAL BIOFEEDBACK

The second major biofeedback approach to the treatment of hypertension has been so-called *thermal biofeedback*. In this procedure, patients are taught to warm certain skin surface areas (usually hands and sometimes feet) through the use of biofeedback. The warming is thought to occur primarily through peripheral vasodilation.

This form of biofeedback has been used for migraine headaches for over 15 years (Blanchard & Andrasik, 1982), and for Raynaud's disease for almost a comparable period of time (Freedman 1987). In both of these classes of disorder (vascular headache and peripheral vascular disease) thermal biofeedback has come to be an accepted alternative or adjunct to drug treatment (Blanchard & Andrasik, 1985; Freedman, 1987).

Recently, uncontrolled reports from the Menninger Foundation (Green, Green, & Norris, 1979; Fahrion et al., 1986) have claimed that thermal biofeedback can be of great value in treating essential hypertension. For example, in one large-scale, uncontrolled series of 61 patients (42 on medication at the start of treatment, 19 who were not medicated), 44 patients (72%) were judged completely successful by either having eliminated all antihypertensive medication ($n = 29$) while BP was below 140/90 or, for the initially unmedicated patients, having BP below 140/90. Only 6 were failures, while the remaining 11 showed either some BP reduction or appreciable reduction in medication. These are stronger results than have been reported for any other stress-management procedure.

In the treatment of hypertension, thermal biofeedback has been hypothesized to work by indirectly inhibiting peripheral sympathetic nervous system activity (Dalessio et al., 1979; Fahrion et al., 1986). More specifically, it has been hypothesized that for the hands (and/or feet) to become warm, there must be dilation of the arteriolae and capillaries of the extremities. For this vasodilation to occur, there must be a reduction of so-called sympathetic tone or peripheral sympathetic nervous system activity. This hand warming is seen as an indirect measure, or indication, of reduced sympathetic outflow, which leads to a reduction in BP. (We have preliminary data indicating a reduction in circulating plasma norepinephrine in hypertensives successfully treated by thermal biofeedback or relaxation training.)

In the Menninger treatment package, there is also brief relaxation via frontal EMG biofeedback, a great deal of attention to deep diaphragmatic breathing, and thermal biofeedback for hand warming and then for foot warming.

SUNY-AMC Hypertension Project
Results

As mentioned earlier, we have conducted a moderate-sized controlled comparison of thermal biofeedback with PMR in patients whose BP was controlled on two antihypertensive medications (Blanchard et al., 1984, 1986). We have also conducted a smaller scale comparison of thermal biofeedback to AT in unmedicated patients whose BPs were in the mild hypertensive range (Blanchard et al., 1987).

With regard to the initial study, we found for thermal biofeedback relatively good initial success on the clinical endpoint of being off the second-stage drug for 2 months while BP remained under control (64.9%) versus 26.5% for those receiving PMR ($\chi^2(1) = 10.50, p < .005$). At one year, 35.1% of patients treated with thermal biofeedback were still successfully off the second-stage drug.

In Table 5–3 are BP results from 3 groups from the comparison to PMR: (a) patients treated while on 2 drugs; (b) patients treated after being withdrawn from the second stage drug; and (c) a set of early relaxation failures who were crossed over to thermal biofeedback. Also

Table 5-3. Author's Results with Thermal Biofeedback Treatment of Hypertension

Condition	n		Pretreatment	Posttreatment	t	p
Treated while on 2 drugs	17	SBP	142.6	130.5	4.51	<.001
(16 sessions, hand warming		DBP	86.4	81.5	2.23	.041
only)						
Withdrawn from 2nd drug,	10	SBP	145.4	140.7	1.13	ns
then treated (16 sessions,		DBP	90.5	86.7	5.12	<.001
hand warming)						
Relaxation failures, treated on	12	SBP	125.9	121.2	2.74	.019
2 drugs (16 sessions, hand		DBP	86.9	83.5	2.48	.031
warming)						
Unmedicated (20 sessions,	12	SBP	131.8	128.0	1.03	ns
hand and foot warming)		DBP	94.8	86.2	2.57	.02

in the table are our results (d) from the study with unmedicated mild hypertensives.

As is obvious from Table 5–3, the thermal biofeedback training led consistently to significant reductions in DBP and often to reductions in SBP. While our results, and the uncontrolled results of Fahrion et al. (1986) await replication, we are very enthusiastic about this form of stress management at this time.

SUNY-AMC Thermal Biofeedback Protocol

While our major study (Blanchard et al., 1986) in this area was conducted on patients who entered with BP controlled on two antihypertensive medications and used primarily hand warming, rather than the combination of hand warming and the foot warming, we have come to believe that the combination is a better overall strategy. Thus the training protocol to be described is an amalgam of our two efforts. A session by session outline is contained in Table 5–4.

First Session

We assume that initial intake (history taking, BP measurement) and assessment (psychological testing, psychophysiological testing) have been completed earlier. Thus this represents the first treatment session. The initial part of the first session is devoted to giving the patient an explanation and rationale for the treatment procedures.

Table 5-4. Session-by-Session Outline for Thermal Biofeedback Training

Session No.	Approximate length	Trainer present or absent	Content
1	65 minutes	Present	Treatment rationale; biofeedback explanation; explanation of autogenic phrases; verbal feedback only of hand warming; explanation of home practice
2	60 minutes	Present	Trainer reads autogenic phrases; feedback available for hand warming
3–8	50 minutes	Absent	Feedback training for hand warming
9	50 minutes	Absent	Introduce bidirectional control of hand temperature; feedback training for hand warming
10–11	50 minutes	Absent	Bidirectional control feedback training
12	55 minutes	Absent except at end	Bidirectional control feedback training; explanation of foot warming
13–16	50 minutes	Absent	Feedback training for foot warming

We recommend taking the patient's BP about 5 minutes into the session and again at the end of the formal training portion.

Verbatim rationale:

This research is designed to investigate nondrug treatment for hypertension or high blood pressure. There are several key assumptions in this research which we would like to share with you.

1. The most basic assumption is that psychological events, or things, can affect physiological events, or things. For instance, most people have blushed or have seen someone blush. In this situation case, a set of circumstances, usually words, leads to the sudden dilation of the tiny blood vessels in the face. It is mediated by the interpretation that the blushing individual puts on the words or circumstances.
2. The second basic assumption is that the level of one's blood pressure can be changed or increased by stress—either physical stress such as exertion or sudden exposure to cold, or by psychological stress.
3. Our third assumption—and this one is reasonably well supported by other research findings—is that various kinds of relaxation training can lead to lowered blood pressure.

The procedures we will be using to help you learn to control your blood pressure are called *biofeedback*. Biofeedback is a process that takes place in a special kind of environment, an electronic environment. It is designed to help you gain control of bodily responses that are not ordinarily thought of as being under voluntary control. More specifically, there is a device for detecting very small changes in temperature called a *thermistor*, which will be attached to your finger. So we first detect and *amplify* the biological response. Second, we convert this response to an easily understood form, such as a visual display or an auditory display. Third, we feed this information back to you: so that in this feedback loop you can gain control of your body's responses. Then eventually you can learn what leads to a change in the response.

You would undoubtedly be aware of a change in your hand temperature of say, 5 degrees, but you might not notice a change of 5 tenths of a degree. In this particular case we can detect changes in finger temperature of 1 tenth of a degree with the machine. With the external feedback, you can learn to detect and then control very small changes in temperature. So that is what the *biofeedback* is about.

Now let me try to explain why warming your hands should help your blood pressure. There are two parts to your nervous system: the voluntary part that controls all of your movements and all of your senses, and the involuntary or automatic part of your nervous system that regulates most of your bodily responses, such as how fast your heart beats or the level of your blood pressure, etc.

This automatic part of your nervous system is called the autonomic nervous system. One of its main parts is called the sympathetic nervous system, and it is involved in helping the body prepare for emergencies. You have probably heard of the so-called fight-or-flight response, which is a set of automatic bodily responses to perceived threat —increased blood flow to the major muscles from increased heart rate and blood pressure, and a constriction of the tiny blood vessels in the body's surface. This is a set of responses preparing the body, literally, to fight or to flee.

Biofeedback is designed to help you gain some degree of voluntary control over the autonomic or automatic nervous system. The ultimate goal of this training is for you to be able to shut off, or dampen down, the level of sympathetic nervous system activity, or arousal, particularly when you are aroused for no adaptive reason.

With increased arousal, the tiny blood vessels in your hands and feet constrict or close down. This leads to a cooling of the skin-surface temperature. If you can reverse this process—that is, if you can warm your hands, and later your feet—you are dilating, or opening up, the tiny blood vessels and hence are reducing the level of sympathetic arousal. Thus, we are using hand temperature as a means of detecting level of sympathetic arousal.

Also, as the peripheral blood vessels dilate and sympathetic arousal decreases, blood pressure decreases because there is less resistance to flow or circulation. This action is part of what the second-stage blood-pressure medication you are on is doing. Thus we hope to substitute a nondrug therapy for at least one of your drugs.

The way you "talk to" your autonomic nervous system is primarily through images and sensations and feelings.

For instance, if I have you think about a fresh juicy lemon, and imagine it, all nice and yellow, try to picture it . . . now imagine slicing it in half and smelling the lemon odor and seeing the juicy inside . . . and think of what it tastes like . . . does your mouth begin to water slightly?

This is an example of imagery stimulating a part of the autonomic nervous system. We have some similar "language" that helps some individuals learn to warm their hands, and I will go through that with you during the session.

Next say to the patient:

You probably want to ask how you are supposed to warm your hands. Unfortunately I cannot give you a specific answer. Instead we can put you in a situation, within our biofeedback loop, where you can discover what method will work for you. In the final analysis, however, you will need to discover for yourself what works for you—what kinds of self-instructions or images or thoughts help you relax and become warm.

Procedures. Show the patient the thermistor and explain that it is the device for detecting skin temperature. Attach the thermistor to the ventral surface of the last digit of the index finger of the nondominant hand. (Be careful not to cut off circulation to the fingertip with the tape or velcro band. Interference with circulation makes it hard for the patient to warm the area.)

Explain to the patient that the session will have 4 parts:

1. Adaptation and baseline during which the patient is to sit quietly.
2. An initial attempt at self-control without feedback.
3. The actual feedback training portion of the session, which lasts about 20 minutes.
4. A second attempt at self-control without feedback.

Actual phase timing should be as follows:

Adaptation: 10 minutes
In-session baseline: 5 minutes
Self-control 1: 5 minutes
Feedback training: 20 minutes
Self-control 2: 5 minutes

For the first session only, the feedback display should not be available to the patient but should be visible to the trainer.

At the beginning of the feedback-training phase, *tell the patient*:

There are *three general parts of the procedure*:
1. *Letting* yourself become *relaxed* in a *passive way*.
2. Regular, diaphragmatic *breathing*.
(Have the patient check his or her breathing by hand on abdomen. The patient should feel rise and fall against the hand as he breathes. If not, work with this until the patient can get it right and then *strongly* suggest regular, brief (1 to 2 minutes) practice of deep, diaphragmatic breathing several times per day.)
3. Allowing or letting your hands become warm. (Again a passive-volitional idea of letting the response occur rather than forcing it.) Acknowledge that this can be difficult at first.

Next explain the autogenic phrases:

> One possible way for you to warm your hands consists of using so-called autogenic phrases. These are a very specific set of self-instructions. I will say a phrase, using the first person. You should then repeat the phrase mentally to yourself. As you repeat it to yourself, you should try to have the experience you are describing. Now close your eyes as I read the phrases.

The autogenic phrases we have used are shown in Table 5–5.

Allow 10 to 15 seconds between phrases.

Periodically tell the patient how his hand temperature is changing, especially if it increases: "that's good, you've increased a tenth of a degree" (or two tenths of a degree, etc.).

If there is a steady decrease, do not mention it early. However, if the whole session shows a downward trend, tell the person: "Well, you have control of part of the temperature response in that you can make it go down. Now let's see if you can make it go in the other direction."

Be sure the room is warm.

At end of session:

1. Give patient self-report form to fill out.
2. Then give the patient the pretreatment rationale questionnaire to fill out.
3. Then give patient copy of autogenic phrases and a few self-report forms to fill out when he practices the hand-warming technique at home. Remind the patient to bring these back at the next session.

Table 5-5. Autogenic Phrases

---

1. I feel quiet.
2. I am beginning to feel quite relaxed.
3. My feet feel heavy and relaxed.
4. My ankles, my knees, and my hips feel heavy, relaxed, and comfortable.
5. My solar plexus, and the whole central portion of my body, feel relaxed and quiet.
6. My hands, my arms, and my shoulders, feel heavy, relaxed, and comfortable.
7. My neck, my jaws, and my forehead feel relaxed. They feel comfortable and smooth.
8. My whole body feels quiet, heavy, comfortable, and relaxed.
9. (Now go back through the sequence on your own.)
10. I am quite relaxed.
11. My arms and hands are heavy and warm.
12. I feel quite quiet.
13. My whole body is relaxed and my hands are warm, relaxed, and warm.
14. My hands are warm.
15. Warmth is flowing into my hands; they are warm, warm.
16. I can feel the warmth flowing down my arms into my hands.
17. My hands are warm—relaxed and warm.
18. (Now go back through the sequence on your own.)

Home practice:

4. Give patient thermometer or other home-practice thermal device for home practice and explain how to use it.
5. Show patient how to tape to nondominant index finger, being careful not to tape all around the finger (which will cut off circulation).
6. Strongly urge at least one practice per day for 20 minutes; two practices would be better. For home practice, the patient should select a comfortable, quiet, relaxed, warm setting.
7. The patient should use autogenic phrases, regular diaphragmatic breathing, and the thermometer.

Remind the patient that the wording of the autogenic phrases does not have to be exactly the same.

Make two manual determinations of BP, beginning of session and at the end of the feedback training.

Second Session

1. Prior to this session, collect the patient's self-report sheets and inquire as to practice efforts at home. Record in the progress notes any special difficulties the patient reports.
2. Again for this session, obtain the adaptation and in-session baseline measures as usual.
3. After the baseline, activate the visual-feedback display only, and set the feedback display at a level sensitive enough to be reinforcing for the patient but insensitive enough so that you will not have to leave the subject room during the session to re-center the meter. Before you enter the room, center the meter.
4. Enter the subject room and remind the subject of the idea of passive volition. Place the meter in such a way that it is visible to both the subject and yourself. Suggest to the subject that you will again read through the autogenic phrases and that she or he may want to occasionally open her eyes to check progress in warming the hands by glancing at the meter. Explain that deflection to the right indicates warming, and so forth.
5. Read through the phrases and have the patient repeat them to herself as during the first session.
   a. If the meter indicates hand warming during the session, call this to the patient's attention and reinforce her success.
   b. If her hand temperature drops and she seems distracted by this, assure her that this is a normal initial reaction and suggest that she focus on the phrases and deep diaphragmatic breathing—and check on the subject's hand temperature only in passing.

6. Remember to measure BP at start of session and at end of Self-control 2.

Sessions Three through Eight

1. Prior to Sessions 3 and 4, collect the subject's self-report sheets. For subsequent sessions collect diary data and immediately record the information on diary-data-reduction sheets.
2. At Session 3, explain to the subject that you will not remain in the same room. Explain the use of the audio feedback. (Explain that increase in hand temperature will correspond to *decrease* in frequency or pitch.) Also indicate to the subject that she or he may use the autogenic phrases as one way to help warm the hands, but that she or he may also want to experiment with other mental techniques that might work for her. Tell her that, even though you will be in constant voice contact with her via the intercom, you will generally speak to her only to indicate the beginning and end of each phase, and to tell her when you are adjusting the feedback meter to re-center it after her temperature is outside the range of the meter.
3. For all subsequent sessions obtain adaptation in the usual manner, then:
   (a) a 5-minute baseline period
   (b) a 5-minute self-control period (indicate to the patient over the intercom that you would like to attempt to warm her hands without the use of the feedback for a few minutes)
   (c) a 20-minute feedback period, and
   (d) a final 5-minute self-control period.
4. (a) During the actual feedback, set the Med Associate ANL 410 sensitivity to 1 or 2 (you may be able to decrease sensitivity to 3 or 4 during later sessions if the patient's hand temperature starts to change significantly, requiring frequent adjustments).
   (b) Set the Med Associate ANL-910 (audio) to a sensitivity of about 5 or 6 and the volume very low (just high enough to be audible over the intercom).
5. After the session be sure to inquire as to whether the patient has a preference regarding the two kinds of feedback display. During subsequent sessions, you may use either or both audio and visual feedback as per the patient's preference.
6. Reminders:
   (a) Be sure to take sitting BP and pulse prior to and after each session.
   (b) Record room temperature on the tape for *all* feedback sessions.
   (c) Encourage regular home practice and BP recording.

Sessions Nine through Twelve:
Bidirectional Training

In our experience most patients begin to show temperature readings in the mid-90s by the sixth or seventh session. In these next four sessions, we seek to consolidate the patient's degree of control by having the patient try bidirectional control of hand temperature.

The patient is told that after he or she reaches 94°F (if using a digital feedback display), you will want him to try to cool his hand by 2 or 3 degrees and then rewarm it. If using an analog display, the trainer should indicate when the patient should begin lowering temperature and then rewarming. The rewarming may prove especially difficult for some patients. Be supportive so they do not become discouraged.

Session Twelve Note

At the end of this session tell the patient that you will begin training in foot warming at the next session. Demonstrate to the patient by taking off your own shoe and sock where the thermistor will be placed. (On the bottom of the great toe.)

Thus, warn the patient to come prepared for this at the next session. For women, have them come without nylon stockings or have them remove the stockings before the session.

Sessions Thirteen through Sixteen:
Foot Warming

At the beginning of this session explain to the patient that he or she will be trying to warm his feet for the next four sessions. The reason for this is to bring about improved vascular and sympathetic nervous system control in the lower extremities (legs).

The session proceeds as if it were a hand-warming session.

Remind the patient that he may have some difficulty at first but that he should again use whatever strategies worked for his hands.

Tell the patient to continue the home practice of hand warming. The patient could also try foot warming at a separate home-practice session if he wants to.

If you have the ability to monitor two temperature channels, you should continue to monitor hand temperature during the foot-warming sessions.

COMMENTS AND CLINICAL HINTS

Number and Spacing of Sessions

As we noted earlier, we have used training regimens of both 16 and 20 sessions. We would recommend contracting with the patient for at least 16 sessions with the possibility of extending to 20 sessions. If you go beyond 16 sessions, these additional sessions should probably be devoted to foot warming. It is not clear at this time whether it is the number of sessions or number of weeks in training that are critical or whether it is rather the degree of temperature control obtained.

We recommend at least two sessions per week. There are no data on session spacing, only clinical judgment. We also strongly recommend at least a day in between sessions.

Although we believe the order of the training tasks presented in Table 5–4 makes sense, we are not sure that the distribution of sessions to the three tasks (50% to hand warming, 25% to bidirectional control, 25% to foot warming) is optimal. It represents the one we have used. It could be that more sessions on foot warming would be beneficial.

Group Treatment

We have found that thermal biofeedback training can readily be accomplished in a small group setting with each patient having access to his own biofeedback device. One should caution the patients *against* competing with each other in, for example, their degree of hand warming, because active striving tends to hamper hand warming.

The Biofeedback Device

There are many commercially available temperature-biofeedback devices. All are based on the use of a thermistor as the sensing device. The thermistor is a small device whose electrical characteristics (namely resistance) change lawfully as a function of temperature. With the appropriate circuitry, one can assess temperature easily to within one-tenth degree Fahrenheit and perhaps to within one or two hundredths of a degree.

The device we use is made by Med Associated (ANL-410); we have also used the Cyborg J-42. In our experience, the commercially available biofeedback devices are every bit as accurate and reliable as most research devices.

Thermal biofeedback devices are typically less expensive than EMG devices.

Feedback modality. We recommend that both visual and auditory feedback displays be available for the patient. In our experience, at least 80% of patients elect a visual display for thermal-biofeedback training. A digital display, which is updated every one to five seconds, rather than a meter also seems effective.

Training schedules. In thermal biofeedback there have been two principal training schedules: (a) continuous trials and (b) discrete trials. Fortunately on this issue there are some empirical data.

Taub and School (1978) recommend discrete training trials of approximately 60 seconds with breaks of from 10 to 15 seconds interspersed. This training schedule arose from their work on the thermal-biofeedback training with paid, normal volunteers. Although the researchers never tested it in a formal experiment, this schedule appears to have been developed empirically through their trying different schedules with subjects over time.

We conducted a pair of experimental studies on this topic. In the first study normal volunteers received four sessions of thermal biofeedback to assist them in warming their hands. Half the subjects received 20 minutes of continuous feedback while the other half received 20 one-minute feedback trials with 10-second rest periods with no feedback interspersed. Both groups showed comparable increases in hand temperature over sessions.

In the second, and more important, study (Andrasik, Pallmeyer, Blanchard, & Attanasio, 1984) patients with vascular headache, either migraine or combined migraine and tension, who had failed to respond to relaxation training, received eight sessions of thermal biofeedback. Half ($n = 8$) received 20 minutes of continuous feedback, while the other half ($n = 8$) received 20 one-minute feedback trials with 10-second rest periods interspersed. In this study the results were clear: As a group, the patients receiving continuous feedback showed modest degrees of acquisition of hand-temperature control, while those receiving discrete trials failed, as a group, to show acquisition. In fact, their performance steadily deteriorated across trials. The two groups were statistically different for each of the last three 5-minute blocks of feedback training.

Two important conclusions emerge from this study: (a) For patients with vascular headache, a continuously available feedback display has a distinct advantage over brief, discrete trials with interspersed rest periods; and (b) one must be cautious about generalizing conclusions on biofeedback training parameters drawn from studies on normal volunteers to patient populations; one must eventually confirm the study on patients.

In a discussion with the patients after this study, we were told that the frequent interruptions caused them "to lose it" and were highly disruptive. We also learned that patients in the continuous display condition did "take breaks" upon occasion, but at their own timing. A compromise might be to use 5-minute feedback trials with 30-second rest periods.

The therapist probably does not have to worry about scheduling rest periods for those patients who have elected to use visual feedback alone. When the patient wants to rest, he or she need only avert the gaze from the feedback display for the desired period. If auditory feedback is selected, then the patient and trainer might want to experiment with moderate-length trials separated by brief rest periods. Based on our experience, the feedback trials should be longer than one minute because many patients report it takes at least this long to re-establish their concentration on the self-regulation task.

Sensor placement. We have used the ventral surface of the index finger of the nondominant hand as the sensor placement. Others (e.g., Fahrion, personal communication) use the little finger. Taub (in Taub & School, 1978) advocates using the web dorsum, that is, the fleshy area of the back of the hand between the thumb and index finger. To the best of our knowledge, no data are available comparing sensor sites.

Site preparation. No special site preparation is necessary other than to have a clean surface. The sensor is usually attached with either paper tape or a velcro band. It is important when tape is used not to encircle the digit completely. The tape should not act as a tourniquet and cut off blood supply.

It is also important to run the cable from the sensor down the finger and attach it to the hand at one point in order to control for what Taub and School (1978) call the "stem effect."

Trainer presence or absence. There are no experimental studies on this factor. Taub recommends the trainer be present and interact with the patient in a "warm, friendly, supportive manner." Although we agree that the trainer should be warm, friendly, and supportive because these are desirable characteristics for any therapist, we have different views on the therapist's presence.

As noted above, we have the therapist present for the first two sessions. After that we train with the therapist absent.

Home Thermal-Biofeedback Devices

For all patients receiving thermal-biofeedback training, we have routinely given them some form of home training device. Initially we used the temperature-sensitive plastic strips that changed color as the finger changed temperature. However, these devices had a rather limited temperature range and the adhesive to hold it to the finger wore out quickly.

For the past few years, we have given patients the small alcohol-in-glass thermometers attached to a cardboard scale, available from the Conscious Living Foundation, Box 9T, Drain, Oregon 97435. These devices can be read easily to within 2°F and with effort to within 1°F.

Explanation to patient of use of home-training thermometer:

> As part of the temperature-biofeedback training, we are going to give you a small, home-training device. This consists of a small thermometer. (Show the patient the device.) Although this device is not as sensitive as the equipment in the laboratory, it is portable and can be used at home. You should tape it to the index finger of one hand. Be careful not to put the tape all the way around the finger. As you are able to begin to warm your hands, the temperature will begin to change.
>
> We would like to practice trying to warm your hands for a few minutes, probably about 5 to 10 minutes, several times per day. We would like for you to practice at least two times a day and more frequently if possible. The purpose is for you to be able to bring about the hand-warming response rapidly. Once you have acquired this hand-warming response, you can practice it regularly to help obtain a sense of relaxation.
>
> To summarize, we want you to begin practicing trying to warm your hands for brief periods at home and to use this little thermometer as a device to assist you. Are there any questions?

There are other more elaborate home-training devices, including the Biotic Band, a temperature-sensitive plastic strip that encircles the finger and registers temperatures within about half a degree. It is fairly expensive. Electronic home-thermal-biofeedback trainers start at about $100 and go up to $800. These devices are commercially available and provide visual feedback as a digital display, usually to within one tenth of a degree, and, in the more expensive models, auditory feedback as well.

We strongly advocate regular home practice of the hand-warming response and of relaxation exercises.

Other clinical hints. As we mentioned earlier, a phenomenon that frequently occurs early in thermal-biofeedback training is that *when a patient tries very hard to warm his or her hands, the hands grow cooler and temperature drops*. In fact, one can almost predict this phenomenon for very achievement-oriented individuals. For such patients, we have found it useful to predict this phenomenon to them; that is, after trying to explain the idea of passive volition, or letting a response occur in a passive, nonstriving fashion, we might suggest that the patient will probably try very hard to warm the hands and experience the cooling. After this occurs, the patient then seems to be more willing to listen.

We suggest to patients that they view the biofeedback situation as a laboratory in which they can experiment with different techniques to see what strategy helps them warm their hands. They are, of course, given one explicit strategy, the autogenic phrases. We also suggest both imagery related to relaxation and imagery related to warmth (such as sitting in front of fire in a fireplace or lying on the beach in the warm sun).

One finds some number of hypertensive patients who begin training with relatively warm hands, say above 92°F. These patients often have difficulty achieving a great deal of warming. We explain to these patients that one cannot expect a great deal of warming for someone whose hands start off so warm. We also suggest they try alternatively warming and cooling the hands within the session to show that they have gained some degree of control.

Minimal-therapist-contact Treatment

We have had very good success treating vascular headache with a largely home-based, self-administered treatment program combining PMR and thermal biofeedback (Jurish, Blanchard, et al., 1983; Blanchard et al., 1985). Reasoning by analogy, we have recently evaluated a similar thermal-biofeedback-treatment program for hypertension (Blanchard et al., 1987 in press).

In this study we compared our standard 16-session, individually administered, clinic-based regimen to a new 5-session program that was largely self-administered and home-based. The first 3 sessions were the same as those described earlier in this chapter. Then patients were seen at 3-week intervals. They were given electronic thermal trainers to use at home. Nine patients with BP controlled on two drugs took part in each regimen.

Results clearly favored the clinic-based program, with 5 of 9 subjects being successfully withdrawn from the second-stage drug, while only 1 of 9 was successful in the home-based program ($p = .05$). In fact, we discontinued the study early because the patients in the home-based program did so poorly. It seemed unethical to continue it further.

Thus, at this point we recommend strongly *against* a minimal-therapist-contact thermal-biofeedback program for hypertension.

Booster Treatments

In our major comparison of thermal biofeedback to PMR (Blanchard et al., 1986), we evaluated during the one-year follow-up the effects of giving patients who had been successfully withdrawn from the second-stage medication monthly booster treatments. In our work with chronic headache (Andrasik et al., 1984) we had found a trend for booster treatment to help with vascular headache.

We found a similar trend ($p < .14$) for booster treatment with thermal biofeedback to help hypertensives stay off the second-stage drug. Thus, at this point we strongly recommend a program of regular booster treatments in the clinic in addition to urging patients to continue regular home practice.

FRONTAL EMG BIOFEEDBACK

A last form of biofeedback which has been used as a treatment of hypertension is called frontal EMG (electromyogram) biofeedback. This procedure was developed by Budzynski and Stoyva (Budzynski & Stoyva, 1969; Budzynski, Stoyva & Adler, 1970) and used initially for the treatment of tension headache. It is still considered the standard biofeedback treatment for tension headache (Budzynski, 1978; Blanchard & Andrasik, 1982).

Since that time, its value as a generalized relaxation procedure (Stoyva & Budzynski, 1974) has been touted and it has been used to treat insomnia, chronic anxiety, and other disorders (Surwit & Keefe, 1978).

Thus, the rationale for use of frontal EMG biofeedback with hypertension is that, through the relaxing of the muscles of the face, scalp and neck, one can achieve a very deep overall state of relaxation. Some believe that use of frontal EMG biofeedback will lead both to a deeper state of relaxation and to one achieved more rapidly. This relaxed state would then have beneficial effects on BP in the same manner as hypothesized earlier in the chapter.

There have been at least two controlled studies that evaluated frontal EMG biofeedback as a treatment for hypertension, one from our laboratory (Blanchard et al., 1979) and one other (Surwit, Shapiro, & Good, 1978). The results from these two studies are given in Table 5–6.

These two studies show relatively little effect of frontal EMG

Table 5-6. Controlled Evaluations of Frontal EMG Biofeedback as a Treatment of BP

Study	Conditions	N	Pretreatment BP		Posttreatment BP		Follow-up BP (6 weeks)	
			SBP	DBP	SBP	DBP	SBP	DBP
Blanchard et al., (1979a)	Frontal EMG biofeedback	10	147	96	149	96	150	94
	Self-relaxation	10	148	88	139	83	144	87
Surwit et al., (1978)	Frontal EMG biofeedback	8	136	—	144	—	136	—
	Relaxation	8	141	—	136	—	135	—

biofeedback on BP despite regimens of 12 and 8 sessions, respectively, and significant reductions in EMG levels. *On the basis of our experience, and that of Surwit et al. (1978), we do not recommend this as a treatment for hypertension.* We should note, however, that McGrady et al. (1981) found positive results with EMG biofeedback-assisted relaxation for hypertensives in an uncontrolled study.

SUNY-ALBANY PROTOCOL FOR FRONTAL EMG BIOFEEDBACK

Despite the recommendation given above, we will describe our protocol for frontal EMG biofeedback.

First Session

An important introductory part of the biofeedback treatment of hypertension, or for that matter, of any psychological treatment of any problem, is to provide the patient with both an explanation of the treatment procedures and a convincing rationale for its use with the patient's presenting problem. These introductory remarks serve at least two purposes: first, they enable the patient to understand the treatment procedures and thus to become an active participant in his own treatment rather than a passive recipient of therapy; second, they serve a motivational function of giving the patient a moderately positive expectancy of success. Research in our laboratory (Shaw & Blanchard, 1983) has shown that positive expectancies lead to greater clinical improvement mediated by more active efforts on the part of the patient to follow instructions outside of the clinic.

Our patients are given the following introduction:

As we discussed at our last session, today we are going to begin the treatment of your hypertension through the use of biofeedback training.

Let me first tell you a little something about biofeedback training. The main idea involved is to help you to learn how to control certain physiological responses. In your particular case, we want you to learn how to relax the muscles of your forehead, scalp, and face using purely mental means.

Numerous clinics and laboratories have shown on an individual basis that teaching people to control the forehead muscles, and especially how to really relax these muscles, can have a very beneficial effect on hypertension.

There are three basic parts to biofeedback: First, we need an electronic gadget to detect very small changes in a particular response—changes so small that you ordinarily cannot detect them. In this case it is very small changes in muscle tension in your forehead. These sensors detect the levels of muscle tension. (Show forehead electrodes to the patient.) It will be necessary for me to clean the skin of your forehead very well so that we get a good signal.

Second, we need to be able to convert these changes to a signal you can easily process. We do this electronically, also.

Finally, we feed this information back to you (hence, biofeedback). For this purpose we will use this speaker. We have several different kinds of auditory feedback and will let you try different ones to see which works best for you. For example, the pitch of the tone may go up or down as you become more tense or more relaxed. Or we may have the tone go off as you relax your forehead below a certain tension level. Or there may be a series of clicks with faster clicks, meaning increasing tension—and slower clicks, meaning increasing relaxation.

There are two important parts of learning to control a response: First, you can use the biofeedback situation as your own laboratory in which you can discover what strategies, tactics, or maneuvers work for you. Thus, we encouarge you to experiment, to try ideas or images you think might work for you.

Second, and very important, is to let the response occur, to be somewhat passive. If you try to force it, to make your forehead less tense, you may become more tense as you try. So remember to relax and let your forehead and your body become more relaxed.

Questions?

The session will have four parts: (a) a brief period while we adjust the equipment to get stable readings, (b) a brief period during which we will ask you to try to relax your forehead without feedback, (c) the feedback training for 20 minutes, and (d) a brief period during which we will ask you to see how well you can maintain control.

The intercom will be open at all times.

Questions?

As noted in the explanation give to patients, our biofeedback training sessions are divided into several phases. (We use the same phases and phase length for frontal EMG biofeedback and for thermal biofeedback, discussed earlier in this chapter.)

The phases and their respective lengths are:

1. Adaptation: 10–15 minutes
2. In-session baseline: 5 minutes
3. Self-control 1: 5 minutes
4. Feedback training: 20 minutes
5. Self-control 2: 5 minutes

Thus, when one adds time for attaching and removing sensors, collecting diary data, and checking on progress and relaxation practice, our average biofeedback training session runs for about 50 minutes.

Clinical Hints

There are many clinical or practical issues to consider in the application of frontal EMG biofeedback training. On some of these issues there are research data to guide clinical practice whereas on other issues we have only our own clinical judgment. On the next few pages we address these issues.

The biofeedback device. There are numerous EMG biofeedback devices commercially available today. Because of the idiosyncrasies of our clinical research operation, we have used none of the commercially available devices. Instead we have used a Grass Instrument Company Model 7 polygraph and Med Associates programming modules. In our opinion, one certainly does not need the research-grade equipment we have used for clinical work. To be a good biofeedback device for research, the device should be reliable, accurate, and able to provide a permanent record of the physiological activity monitored. It is our impression that some of the commercially available EMG biofeedback devices are adequate for research purposes.

The EMG signal has an estimated frequency range (or *bandpass*) of approximately from 1 to 1000 Hz. In our research, we have used a Grass 7-P3 Preamplifier with a bandpass of from 3 to 300 Hz. Most commercially available EMG biofeedback devices have a bandpass of from 100 to 200 Hz. This latter situation leads to the unfortunate electronic elimination of much of the EMG signal by these devices.

Feedback modality. Although most EMG biofeedback devices have both auditory and visual feedback displays available, it has become the almost universal custom to use auditory feedback when giving feedback from the frontal placement. Part of the reason for this choice is that patients can keep their eyes closed with auditory feedback, thus minimizing eye-movement artifacts in the signal. Moreover, both clinical opinion and unpublished data on normals from our laboratory have shown that individuals obtain lower EMG levels with auditory as opposed to visual feedback.

Most devices offer a variety of auditory feedback signals including a binary signal in which a tone goes off as the EMG level drops below a fixed level and an analog signal in which the pitch of a tone decreases as EMG level decreases. Another popular form of feedback is a click rate. Auditory clicks are provided at a rate proportional to EMG level such that a lower rate of clicks represents a decreased EMG level.

In our work we have made all three of these auditory modalities available to patients and have let them decide which they prefer. We would recommend this feedback-display sampling as a routine practice for the clinician to try with patients.

Training schedules. As discussed earlier under thermal biofeedback, it is possible to subdivide the actual biofeedback training portion of a treatment session in many ways. Unpublished data from our laboratory comparing 20 minutes of continuously available EMG feedback to 20 one-minute discrete trials with 10-second intervals between trials tended to show an advantage for the continuously available feedback. In fact, some patients complained that the short trials and frequent interruptions were disruptive.

It is our impression that some patients take breaks, that is, they work at the task for a while and then stop concentrating for a while. You might try a training schedule of 5-minute feedback trials with 30-second breaks. We have no data on this schedule, however.

Presence or absence of the therapist. In our frontal EMG biofeedback training, we have always conducted sessions with the therapist absent from the patient chamber beginning with the first session. (In our thermal biofeedback training we use a slightly different format, see section earlier in this chapter.) The therapist is, of course, in constant voice contact by intercom with the patient and can observe the patient through a one-way glass.

There is certainly no uniform opinion on this issue, as evidenced by the comments by Steiner and Dince (1981) favoring therapist presence. Fortunately, there are empirical data available on this issue from an excellent study by Borgeat, Hade, Larouche, and Bedwani (1980). Using tension and combined-tension-and-migraine patients, they compared the effects of therapist presence to therapist absence. In the therapist-present condition, "the therapist was physically present with the patient, coaching, encouraging, providing information about overall progress, and looking with the patient for causes of poor performance." Results showed consistently higher frontal EMG levels in the therapist-present condition with the results being statistically significant ($p < .2$) in baseline and approaching significance ($p < .10$) in the feedback and what would be self-control 1 and 2 conditions. Moreover, patients were switched at midtraining (after six sessions) from one condition to the other. Significantly more patients (six of eight) showed poorer performance after switching from therapist-absent to therapist-present than in the therapist-present to therapist-absent order (one of eight; $p < .02$). Headache reduction was equivalent for the two conditions. This study is especially important because it was done with patients under clinical conditions.

Dumouchel (personal communication, 1983) also has unpublished data showing that some patients do more poorly at any biofeedback training task with the therapist present than with the therapist absent.

Thus, we would recommend conducting frontal EMG biofeedback training with the therapist absent. However, because this may not be possible with some equipment and in some laboratory set-ups, we would recommend that the therapist refrain from active coaching if remaining in the room with the patient.

Electrode-site preparation. In accordance with most psychophysiological recording recommendations, we routinely prepare the site for the sensors by scrubbing the skin lightly with a mild abrasive such as Brasivol and then cleaning fine debris with an alcohol wipe (cotton or gauze pad soaked in isopropanol alcohol). At a minimum, one should clean the site thoroughly with an alcohol wipe.

One should also be sure to clean the electrode cups between uses so as to have a uniform contact medium in the recording.

Electrode placement. According to the Biofeedback Society of America's Task Force Report on the treatment of tension headache (Budzynski, 1978), the standard electrode placement for the EMG biofeedback treatment of tension headache is a frontal one, hence the term frontal EMG biofeedback. This placement, described in Lippold (1967), was the one used by Budzynski and his associates in their pioneering work in this field (Budzynski et al., 1970). The two active electrodes are located on the forehead, one approximately one inch above each eyebrow, centered on the eye. The ground electrode is centered between these two active electrodes. We have used this placement in all of our EMG biofeedback treatments of hypertensive patients.

EMG Biofeedback-training Tips

We strongly advocate telling the patient to experiment with the biofeedback situation to learn which strategies work for him. Thus, we routinely suggest to patients that they test the responsiveness of the biofeedback by deliberately tensing their forehead for a few moments in order to hear what happens to the feedback display.

If the patient is having difficulty with EMG biofeedback training, there are two things one can try: (a) Intersperse some bidirectional control trials. Throughout most training sessions, the patient has a single goal of trying to lower frontal EMG level. In the bidirectional-control procedure, the patient is asked to increase and then decrease frontal EMG for periods of about 30 seconds. Because most patients can suceed at increasing EMG levels, they experience some success and the therapist can encourage them by noting that the patient can exert some control. Furthermore, a muscle group may become more relaxed than usual after being deliberately tensed. (b) Given the overall therapeutic value of a success experience at bodily control for tension-headache patients demonstrated by Holroyd et al. (1984), it is sometimes advantageous to change surreptitiously a sensitivity setting or a level indicator on the biofeedback device so that, by the feedback received, the patient is led to believe that he or she is becoming successful at the task. This tactic should probably be reserved for later sessions when the patient has become fairly discouraged. It seems to have a strong motivating effect on the patient.

Chapter 6

Exercise as a Treatment for Hypertension

The present chapter focuses on the second important behavioral risk factor connected with elevated blood pressure, physical inactivity, and its converse, exercise. In this discussion we will present the evidence for, and the methods of, employing exercise ... the nondrug therapy for the hypertensive. The support for the use of exercise in the behavioral treatment of hypertension comes from several directions, including epidemiologic and experimental studies, and from the authors' (JEM, PMD) experience at the Jackson VA Medical Center between 1980 and 1986. We will summarize this evidence in the initial sections of this chapter. Subsequently, we will present and discuss the exercise program we developed in Jackson, step-by-step, including strategies designed to maximize adherence to the physical-activity program.

THE EVIDENCE FOR THE ANTIHYPERTENSIVE EFFECT OF EXERCISE

In one of the earliest reports that exercise may independently exert an antiphypertensive effect, Steinhaus noted in 1933 that athletes and outdoor sportsmen had lower resting blood pressures than did those who were not involved in sports activities (Steinhaus, 1933). In an intriguing clinical study, Morris and Crawford (1958) found on autopsy that hypertensives who had died of various causes exhibited fewer and less severe physiological sequelae of their elevated blood pressure if they had been more physically active. These early suggestive studies were followed by much more carefully controlled and extensive investigations into the relationship between exercise and high blood pressure.

Epidemiologic Studies

Two epidemiologic studies with positive findings were reported in investigations conducted in the late 1960s (Montoye, Metzner, Keller, Johnson, & Epstein, 1972; Gyntelberg, 1974). In these studies, a moderately positive association was established between levels of physical activity and resting blood pressure. Somewhat curiously, prior to these reports, population studies correlating physical activity, fitness levels, and the incidence and severity of hypertension had been relatively mixed (Tipton, 1984; Leon & Blackburn, 1982). Not long after these mildly supportive studies were conducted, an important study was in the works at Harvard.

The Harvard Alumni Studies. In the most recent epidemiologic study looking at hypertension risk and exercise, Paffenbarger and colleagues (Paffenbarger, Wing, Hyde, & Jung, 1983) reported perhaps the best evidence for the importance of regular physical activity to blood pressure control and hypertension risk. A sample of 14,998 male Harvard alumni were followed during the study for 6 to 10 years. These alumni had entered Harvard between 16 and 50 years prior to the study. The findings were clear and striking: The lack of strenuous current exercise, along with body fat and parental hypertension, were all found to independently predict risk of hypertension. Importantly, current and regular vigorous exercise was inversely related to hypertension risk.

Taken together, the epidemiologic findings suggest (though they cannot provide causal proof) that exercise may be an important factor in the avoidance of developing elevated blood pressure. The Harvard alumni study further indicates that the apparent protective aspect of fitness was not due to subject-selection bias, but was indeed related to the *current* practice of regular physical activity, particularly aerobic training.

Clinical Studies of Exercise in Hypertension

Of course, the correlation of current physical activity and blood pressure is not sufficient evidence on which to base a nondrug treatment for controlling hypertension. Thus, it is important at this point to turn to the experimental evidence linking exercise with actual blood-pressure lowering in those with hypertension.

The Morris and Crawford (1958) autopsy study served as an interesting precursor to some of the experimental, prospective clinical investigations. Their findings, along with the earlier epidemiologic studies, did not appear to attract much attention—perhaps because the study came at a time when the antihypertensive medications were being used more extensively (and effectively), and the VA cooperative studies (summarized in Chapter 1) were demonstrating the efficacy of pharmacological agents in modulating the cardiovascular morbidity and mortality associated with uncontrolled blood pressure. In light of the inconsistent findings of the earliest (correlational) exercise/blood-pressure studies and the relative ease of administering high potent antihypertensive medications, it is not too surprising that prior to 1970 few other researchers systematically evaluated exercise as a possible alternative or adjunct to these highly potent pharmacological agents in the management of high blood pressure.

Nonetheless, eight investigations (deVries, 1970; Johnson & Grover, 1967; Hanson & Nedde, 1970; Barry et al., 1966; Boyer & Kasch, 1970; Rudd & Day, 1967; Wilmore, Royce, Girandola, Katch, & Katch, 1970; Kiveloff & Huber, 1971), all conducted between 1966 and 1971, provided some highly suggestive, albeit poorly controlled and somewhat inconsistent, clinical evidence for the antihypertensive effect of exercise.

Fifteen studies (Sannerstedt et al., 1973; Choquette & Ferguson, 1973; Bonanno & Lies, 1984; Ressl, Chrastek & Jandova, 1977; Krotkiewski et al., 1979; Roman, Camuzzi, Villanlon, & Klenner, 1981; Cade et al., 1984; Deplaen & Detry, 1980; Kukkonen, Rauramaa, Voutilainen, & Lansimies, 1982; Nomura et al., 1984; Hagberg et al., 1983; Dubbert, Martin, et al., 1984; Duncan et al., 1985; Martin, Dubbert, & Cushman, 1985) were subsequently conducted over the next 10-to-15-year period with for the most part similarly encouraging results. However, a number of the studies continued to be inadequately controlled, while some even failed to monitor possible confounding variables such as sodium intake and weight change.

In a review of the human experimental literature on the effects of aerobic exercise on blood pressure in hypertension (Martin & Dubbert, 1985), we found that seven of the 16 studies reviewed were uncontrolled evaluations with a combined N of 183, and a mean blood-pressure reduction of -19 mm Hg in systolic blood pressure (SBP) and -14 in diastolic blood pressure (DBP). Three additional studies were partially controlled, in that they employed normotensive exercise controls. These studies had a total N of 68, showing a mean blood-pressure reduction of

Table 6-1. Exercise in Hypertension Studies

Study	Subjects	Exercise	Period	X̄ BP Change (mm Hg)
Controlled Studies				
deVries	66 middle-aged & Geriatric HT Males (X̄ BP 140/76)	Walk, Jog, etc. (30–40 min/3× wk)	7 wk.	−4/−3
Bonnano & Lies	12 HT Males (X̄ BP = 138/92) 8 NTs	Walk/jog (40–55 min/3× wk)	3 mo.	−13* −14*
Deplaen & Detry	6 HT Males & Females (X̄ BP = 169/108)	Walk, Jog, Bike, Calisthenics (60 min/3× wk)	3 mo.	−1 +3
Kukkonen et al.	13 borderline HT (X̄ BP = 145/99)	Walk/Jog, Bike, x-count ski (50′ 3×/wk)	4 mo.	−9* −11*
Nomura et al.	21 mild-moderate HT a) 7 M (X̄ BP = 152/100)	Ergometer 6′/4× day/ 7× wk	3 wk.	−5.8* −9.4*
	b) 14 M & F (X̄ BP = 153/97)	Same as above + salt restriction	3 wk.	−11.4* −8.3*
Hagberg et al.	25 adolescent borderline HT Males & Females (X̄ BP = 137/80)	Jog (40 min/5× wk)	6 mo.	−8* −5*
Dubbert et al.	2 mild HT Males BP = 93 DBP (S1) 96 DBP (S2)	S1: Jog/Ergometer S1: Jog/Swim	3 wk. 10 wk.	−7 DBP −9 DBP
Hagberg et al.	6 Hemodialysis HT Males (X̄ BP = 155/83)	Walk, Jog, Bike, etc. (30 min/3–5× wk)	4 mo.	
Duncan et al.	44 HT Ms (X̄ BP 146/94)	Walk/Jog (60 min/3× wk)	4 mo.	Hi Catech −15.5* (*n* = 18) −8.1* Lo Catech −10.3* (*n* = 26) −6.4*
Martin et al.	10 HT M (X̄ BP = 137/95)	Walk, Jog, Bike (30 min/3–4× wk)	10 wk.	−6.4 −9.6*

*.001 < *p* < .05
a. mean arterial pressure   c. HT = hypertensives
b. estimated from figure   M = males

−15 SBP and −9 DBP. Finally, six studies were better controlled and included hypertensive (wait list/nonexercise) control subjects. Unfortunately, no alternative treatments or attention/placebo controls were included. For these more controlled studies, the weighted mean blood-pressure reduction for the 65 exercised hypertensives was −8 mm Hg SBP and −6 mm Hg DBP. In about half the studies, weight, and even less frequently sodium excretion, were tracked to ensure that changes in these variables did not explain the blood-pressure reduction. Importantly, in three of the six better controlled studies, untreated hypertensive controls exhibited reductions in blood pressure also, with those reductions reaching significance in two of the studies.

Since that earlier review, several more studies have been conducted, including much better controlled studies from the Cooper Institute for Aerobics Research in Dallas (Duncan et al., 1985), and from our laboratory in Jackson (Martin, Dubbert & Cushman, 1985; submitted), and which will be discussed in more detail. Table 6–1 has been provided to illustrate the basic results of the more highly controlled studies that included at least a hypertensive control group, though not necessarily a placebo exercise control (only one study included this).

On the whole, this evidence indicates that, although there were some reports of little or no positive effects of exercise over control conditions, aerobic exercise tends to lower blood pressure across a wide variety of hypertensives, from mild to moderate hypertension, adolescent to geriatric hypertensives, and even hypertensives with advanced-end-organ damage such as renal dialysis patients. Two groups of studies illustrate best the relationship between exercise, fitness, and blood pressure in hypertension and therefore warrant a closer look.

The Cooper Institute for Aerobics Research Studies

Additional supportive evidence for the benefits of exercise in hypertension comes from reports of the 12-year follow-up of more than 6000 men and women seen at the Cooper Clinic in Dallas. Blair and his colleagues (Blair, Goodyear, Gibbons, & Cooper, 1984) found that after adjusting for sex, age, and follow-up interval, men and women showing less physical fitness on a graded exercise test had a relative risk of 1.52 for developing hypertension when compared with highly fit persons who were able to exercise longer at higher workloads.

Subsequently, Duncan and colleagues (Duncan et al., 1985) at the Institute for Aerobics Research compared the effects of an aerobic regimen (60 minutes, three times per week) that was similar to those of the previous studies investigating exercise effects in hypertension (see

Table 6–1), on 56 male hyperadrenergic (elevated plasma catechol-amines) and normoadrenergic hypertensives. A control group of hyper-tensives received only periodic blood pressure checks during the 16-week training period. Changes in DBP associated with the exercise regimen averaged +2.9, −6.4, and −8.1 mm Hg across control, normo-adrenergic and hyperadrenergic subjects. The pattern of changes in SBP across the three groups of subjects was very similar. Pre to post blood pressures and differences between exercised and nonexercised hyper-tensives were statistically significant for both SBP and DBP. A possible mechanism was suggested by the fact that in the hyperadrenergic exercise group, changes in BP were associated with changes in plasma catecholamine values. That is, hypertensive patients showing the highest catecholamine levels initially experienced the largest reductions in blood pressure in conjunction with exercise (−15.5 mm Hg) when compared with the normoadrenergic hypertensives (−10.3 mm Hg). Further, the blood pressure reduction in the hyperadrenergic patients was associated with a significant drop in their catecholamines.

The Jackson Studies

The first of a series of studies conducted by our group at the Jackson VA Medical Center represented an uncontrolled pilot evaluation of the effects of aerobic exercise on mild hypertensives (Martin, Dubbert, Lake, & Burkett, 1982). In this initial study, 10 adult males with unmedicated pressures in the mild hypertensive range (X initial BP = 135/92.3) underwent 10 weeks of twice-weekly aerobic-exercise training in our laboratory, and twice-weekly sessions in the home environment. Exercise consisted of 30 minutes of brisk walking/jogging or bicycle ergometer work at 60% to 75% of aerobic capacity. The results indicated that aerobic exercise was associated with significant ($p < .05$) decreases in both SBP and DBP. Systolic BP dropped a mean of 13.7 mm Hg, whereas DBP fell an average of 9.7 mm Hg.

These blood pressure reductions were not accompanied by any changes in weight or 24-hour sodium values.

In a second, single-subject experiment, we employed hypertensive subjects as their own controls in an experimental, ABAB investigation (Dubbert, Martin, Zimmering, Burkett, Lake, & Cushman, 1984). In this study, two unmedicated adult males with mild hypertension were placed on an exercise regimen including three to five days per week of aerobic walking/jogging, swimming, or bicycle ergometer work. The ABAB withdrawal-reinstatement treatment design was chosen to isolate the specific effects of exercise on diastolic blood pressure, thereby suggesting the functional relationship between exercise and blood pressure levels. In both subjects, regular exercise was discontinued following an initial demonstration of blood pressure change, and diastolic pressure was observed to return to mild hypertensive levels within 5 to 8 weeks after exercise was reduced or discontinued. In the final phase of the study, exercise treatment was reinstated and diastolic blood pressure returned to the normotensive range within 2 or 3 weeks. One subject was followed for a year after he resumed exercising, and his blood pressure remained in the normotensive range despite a small weight gain.

In a subsequent, randomized study (Martin, Dubbert, & Cushman, 1985; submitted), we then attempted to determine if the apparent antihypertensive effect of exercise was due to some other factor, such as expectation/placebo aspects of a general activity program, or if very low-level physical activities could lower blood pressure (perhaps due to some arousal reduction/relaxation or time-out-from-stress phenomenon). In fact, none of the previous studies, controlled or uncontrolled, had used a credible treatment alternative (other than drugs) or placebo group to partial out any nonspecific treatment factors. In our study, we randomly assigned 27 male subjects with mild hypertension (mean baseline BP: 136.6/94.8 mm Hg) to ten weeks of either aerobic training or a placebo control treatment consisting of nonaerobic (less than 60% aerobic capacity) stretching and easy calisthenics. Subjects were unmedicated or had been faded from their medication such that they had been medication free for at least one month. The aerobic regimen consisted of walking, jogging, and/or stationary bicycling for 30 minutes, 4 times per week, at greater than 65% maximal heart rate (this generally averaged 70%). The nonaerobic control regimen consisted of slow calisthenics and stretching for the same duration and frequency but maintaining less than 60% maximal heart rate.

The results of this better controlled study, shown in Table 6–2, were very encouraging. We found that DBP decreased 9.6 mm Hg in the aerobic exercise group but increased 0.8 mm Hg in the placebo control exercise group. Systolic blood pressure (SBP) decreased 6.4 mm Hg in the aerobic group and increased 0.9 mm Hg in the controls. The changes in DBP were statistically significant ($p = .02$), whereas the SBP changes failed to reach significance ($p = .11$). Importantly, these blood pressure changes were not associated with any significant changes in weight, body fat, urinary electrolytes, resting heart rate (HR) or catecholamines.

To further test the reliability of the apparent antihypertensive effect of the aerobic exercise, we then offered the aerobic regimen to the unsuccessful control subjects (similarly to our $N = 2$, ABAB design discussed previously). When the aerobic exercise was performed by the

Table 6-2. Randomized Control Mississippi Study—Exercise Effects in Mild Hypertension[a,b]

	Aerobic Exercise Group (N = 10)	Control Exercise Group (N = 9)
Systolic BP, Pre	136.6 ± 9.4	134.9 ± 5.7
(mm Hg) Post	130.2 ± 10.2	135.8 ± 7.9
Change‡	−6.4 ± 9.1	+0.9 ± 9.7
Diastolic BP, Pre	94.8 ± 4.6	93.7 ± 3.6
(mm Hg) Post	85.2 ± 5.0	94.4 ± 4.3
Change*	−9.6 ± 4.7*	+0.8 ± 6.2*
Resting heart rate, Pre	80.7 ± 8.5	78.8 ± 9.8
(beats/min) Post	72.4 ± 9.4	76.8 ± 10.3
Change‡	−8.3 ± 9.7	−2.4 ± 15.9
Work capacity, Pre[c]	11.2 ± 2.3	9.7 ± 1.7
(METS) Post[c]	13.2 ± 1.8	11.2 ± 1.4
Change‡[d]	+2.0 ± 2.2	+1.5 ± 1.2
Body weight, Pre	90.3 ± 18.0	92.0 ± 15.8
(Kg) Post	89.9 ± 17.0	92.4 ± 16.9
Change‡	−0.4 ± 1.9	+0.4 ± 1.4
Sodium excretion, Pre	235.8 ± 7.4	283.0 ± 137.6
(mEq/24 hrs) Post	202.5 ± 36.3	258.4 ± 101.5
Change‡	−33.4 ± 91.3	−24.6 ± 148.6

[a]Groups were not significantly different ($p < 0.05$) at baseline except where indicated.
[b]Changes from pretreatment to posttreatment were not significantly different ($p < 0.05$) except where indicated.
[c]Groups were significantly different ($p = 0.028$) at pre- and posttreatment.
[d]Both groups showed significant ($p = 0.001$) improvements at posttreatment.
‡Nonsignificant Time × Group Interaction ($p < 0.10$)
*Significant Time × Group Interaction ($p < 0.05$)

control exercise subjects, the results replicated the effects for the original aerobic group. Significant reductions occurred in both DBP (-7.2 mm Hg; $p = .007$) and SBP (-8.1 mm Hg; $p = .005$) of the former control group when the experimental regimen of aerobic exercise was provided.

Thus, our later study constitutes the first placebo-controlled demonstration of the beneficial effects of exercise in hypertension, ruling out nonspecific treatment effects, patient expectations for improvement (credibility ratings were similar for both treatments), as well as time and repeated measurement, as alternative explanations for the improved blood pressures. Importantly, of the 17 subjects who received the 10 weeks of aerobic training (10 randomly assigned originally to aerobic exercise and 7 who received aerobic training after completing the control exercise protocol), 14 achieved DBP levels < 90 mm Hg.

Summary of Exercise Effects in Hypertension Control

Most of the studies reviewed indicate that aerobic exercise can produce a moderate antihypertensive effect of between 5 mm Hg and 15 mm Hg (principally in DBP, though SBP may also decrease significantly) in individuals of all ages with mild to moderate hypertension. Our studies at the Jackson VAMC and those conducted at the Cooper Clinic provide particularly strong evidence that moderately vigorous aerobic activity has the potential of lowering blood pressure in mild hypertensives.

ESTABLISHING AN EXERCISE PROGRAM:

Adherence considerations. Despite the paucity of adequately controlled experimental studies, and the present lack of major clinical trials demonstrating the widespread efficacy of exercise in the longer term control of elevated blood pressure, the present evidence would indicate that at least in select individuals, a systematic program of regular aerobic exercise can serve to independently reduce blood pressure. In the future, more carefully controlled studies are likely to be conducted to further establish the efficacy, durability, dose-response and mechanism(s) of action, appropriate patients for, and generalizability of exercise in the treatment and control of high blood pressure.

On the basis of the evidence reviewed here, and the general appeal of a more natural, health-oriented approach to controlling elevated blood pressure, a number of physicians, health practitioners and hypertensive patients themselves have become proponents of exercise as at least one counterprocedure in the fight to control high blood pressure. We believe that under carefully prescribed and monitored conditions and close medical supervision, it may be appropriate for at least mild hypertensives to engage in a systematic program of aerobic training in an effort to lower blood pressure. Accepting this, one must then turn attention to the second most critical question after "Does it work?" Namely: "Is it possible to get hypertensives to exercise?"

The demonstration of the efficacy of exercise in lowering blood pressure and subsequent prescription by a physician or other health care professional is not sufficient in and of itself to ensure that the exercise will be effectively initiated and maintained. In fact, research suggests that the majority of people who eventually begin an exercise program will stop, often within the first few months (Dishman, 1982; Martin & Dubbert, 1982a, 1982b). Also, adherence is disappointingly low among those enrolled in structured exercise programs for prevention/health enhancement and for rehabilitation following appearance of coronary heart disease (CHD). For example, approximately half of the participants in primary prevention studies will drop out within 3 to 6 months of program entry, whereas for secondary prevention programs, drop-out approaches 50% by about 12 months (Oldridge, 1982; Martin & Dubbert, 1982a). This point is illustrated in a well-controlled study reported by Kentala (1972), who found only 77 out of 298 post-myocardial infarction patients entered a prescribed exercise program. Moreover, 71% of these exercisers dropped out within 5 months, and only 13% continued to exercise through 1 year. Therefore, adherence to exercise regimens is clearly a significant problem. We believe the manner in which exercise programs are established is of paramount importance in determining patient adherence.

Several bodies of research and clinical experience would suggest that it is indeed possible to get basically sedentary individuals, in this case who happen to have hypertension, to exercise on a consistent enough basis to lower their blood pressure (Martin & Dubbert, 1985a). For example, coronary prevention and rehabilitation trials have accrued a large body of information on those individuals and exercise programs found successful in effectively establishing the exercise habit. In addition, a number of experimental studies have suggested techniques that are beneficial in enhancing exercise adoption and continuation. Finally, some approaches developed in our program have been found helpful in shaping and maintaining exercise behavior in sedentary hypertensives and others. Our special attention to these adherence issues when we set up the exercise program for the hypertension studies suggests that it is very possible to get sedentary medical patients to exercise: In fact, 77% of the subjects who were randomized in our study completed the 10-week program, and 100% of those who crossed over to aerobic training following the ineffective control protocol completed the second 10-week program.

In the following sections of the chapter, findings from these three bodies of evidence (primary- and secondary-prevention trials, coronary-rehabilitation studies, and exercise-modification experiments) will be summarized to suggest pathways and pitfalls in approaching the sedentary hypertensive with a prospective exercise treatment regimen. Importantly, this exercise prescription will be similar regardless of whether it is implemented alone or in conjunction with other pharmacological and nonpharmacological procedures.

Exercise-adherence predictors. A wealth of data from coronary-prevention trials and cardiac-rehabilitation programs have provided profiles of the individuals who are most and least likely to initiate and adhere to a systematic exercise program. These studies have been reviewed in several places (Oldridge, 1982; Martin & Dubbert, 1982, 1985; Dishman, 1982) and the interested reader is directed to those sources for further details. Those most likely to succeed with an exercise prescription are nonobese, nonsmoking white-collar workers with active family support and encouragement for exercising, who have higher self-motivation to exercise (this may include having symptoms that might be alleviated or improved by regular exercise). Highest risk drop-out candidates are blue-collar workers who smoke, are overweight and unmotivated, and who have little or no support for the exercise from significant others in the home or work environments.

It is possible that those hypertensives who are poorer risk (in terms of probability of adherence) exercise candidates can be retained in a program if targeted for closer supervision and more gradual increases in exercise intensity and complexity. Such individuals, however, have never been formally identified and given special treatment in an experimental program. Although we would encourage readers, especially those less experienced with highly resistant nonexercisers, to market exercise treatment primarily to those with a lower risk for drop-out, we would also suggest attempting special intervention rather than simply allowing those high-risk patients to drop out.

Exercise-adherence facilitators. Some additional factors that seem to promote initial exercise participation as well as later program adherence pertain to the exercise program itself. For example, retrospective data from cardiovascular treatment and prevention programs strongly suggest that the convenience, location, mode, and topography of the exercise each significantly affect the probability that an individual will participate in exercise.

Most importantly, the *exercise location* must be convenient. That is, it should be either close to work, close to home, or conveniently in between. We actively discourage our clients from joining health spas or programs that require any significant amount of driving or other special preparation. A convenient location increases both the probability that an individual will both make a commitment to participate and then maintain the habit. Seemingly small factors such as difficulty finding parking spaces can have a major negative impact on exercise program attendance and overall adherence.

In fact, the degree of available, active, *social support* or reinforcement for exercise from the home environment has consistently been related to increased exercise adherence. For example, patients with spouses who support their exercise habit are much more likely to have good adherence than those whose spouses are either neutral or negative toward exercising (Andrew et al., 1981). Finally. the amount of social support during exercise is another critical factor in determining exercise adherence (Martin et al., 1984). We tap into both these enhancers by encouraging family members to come to exercise sessions (and to exercise) with their hypertensive significant other, and, as well, to exercise or at least provide praise and support during or after home-exercise participation. For high-risk drop-outs we specifically target the family for this type of co-participation. Finally, long-term adherence can be enhanced for individuals participating in group exercise rather than exercising alone, and so we always encourage (if not organize) clinic and home-exercise groups.

The *mode, or type, of exercise* should also be simple and convenient. For example, most programs stress walking and jogging, as we do, because they can be performed with minimum preparation, cost and equipment, in almost any location, and in all seasons (although some of our northern neighbors have turned by necessity to winter walking in the indoor shopping malls). Also, calisthenics are a poor choice, especially if done when alone and without other easier aerobic exercises such as brisk walking. Most people prefer exercising in groups and will have up to twice the adherence levels than when they try to maintain a lonely exercise regimen.

Finally, how one performs the exercise is of utmost importance to the probability of developing and maintaining the exercise habit. Aerobic *exercise intensity* greater than 85% maximum HR/aerobic capacity, more than 5 times per week, and more than 45 minutes per session is associated with higher drop-out and injury rates. The bulk of the studies with hypertensives has only required a minimum aerobic exercise dose to ensure reductions in blood pressure. Generally, effective exercise regimens for blood pressure modulation consisted of 20 to 30 minutes, 3 times a week, around 70% to 75% maximum HR, of an easy aerobic activity such as brisk walking (more on this in the following sections).

It would be useful at this point to further lay the context for our exercise program for hypertensives by overviewing the literature on experimentally modifying exercise adherence. In setting up our program we relied on this research, including our own studies on exercise adherence, and feel that it would be important for the reader to come to a better understanding of these findings before being led through our systematic exercise format for treating mild hypertension.

Exercise-modification studies. A number of studies have prospectively targeted the modification of exercise adherence in both clinical and, more typically, apparently healthy populations. These interventional studies have been presented and discussed elsewhere (Martin &

Dubbert, 1982; 1985; Dishman, 1982), and will not be reiterated here, except in the way of a summary.

These studies are useful in that they suggest both what does not appear effective (health education alone), as well as the techniques that hold promise (contracting, reinforcement and stimulus-control procedures). On the other hand, they must be interpreted cautiously due to their select populations and limited measurement and design characteristics. Overall, these studies indicate that exercise is a behavior that can be modified using consequent/reinforcement control, stimulus control, and cognitive/self-control techniques. In particular, the use of reinforcement procedures such as contracting and lotteries, praise and social support during exercise, cognitive self-control procedures such as self-contracting and self-reinforcement, individualized and flexible goal setting, and cognitive distraction have all been shown to be effective in increasing exercise adherence-levels 25% to 100% above baseline or control-group levels (Martin & Dubbert, 1982; 1984; 1985; Martin, Dubbert, et al., 1984).

Table 6-3. Borg Rating of Perceived Exertion (RPE) Scale[a]

Rating	Definition
6[*]	
7	"Very, Very Light"
8	
9	"Very Light"
10	
11	"Fairly Light"
12	
13[**]	"Somewhat Hard"
14	
15	"Hard"
16	
17	"Very Hard"
18	
19	"Very, Very Hard"
20[***]	

[*]Corresponds to an average resting HR of 60 beats per min.
[**]Corresponds to an average work (maximum aerobic) capacity of 70%
[***]Corresponds to an average maximum HR of 200 beats per min.
[a]From Borg, G. V. (1970). Perceived exertion as an indicator of somatic stress. *Scandinavian Journal of Rehabilitative Medicine*, 2, 92–98.

Table 6-4. Exercise Enjoyment Scale

Very Unenjoyable	Somewhat Unenjoyable	Neutral	Somewhat Enjoyable	Very Enjoyable
1	2	3	4	5

The Jackson exercise-adherence package. In general, we make ample use of the behavioral techniques of gradual shaping, positive feedback and reinforcement, contracting, and generalization programming. During the laboratory sessions we gradually shape the exercise "duration and intensity" from two 10 to 15 minute periods (separated by a brief, 1 to 2-minute rest break) at 60% maximum HR during the first 1 to 3 weeks, up to a maximum of 30 minutes at 75% to 80% maximum HR by the end of the second month. Depending on their initial fitness level, enjoyment, and perceived and actual exertion levels, as well as their stated desire to move up, we can slow or speed up gradual progression in exercise duration and intensity. Importantly, to assist us in calibrating appropriately comfortable work loads, we carefully track both exertional levels using the Borg Rating of Perceived Exertion (RPE) scale (Borg, 1970), shown in Table 6–3, and our own 5-point exercise-enjoyment scale shown in Table 6–4. We find that an optimal exertional level is between an RPE of 10 and 12 initially, and between 11 and 13 eventually. To enforce our rule of keeping beginning exercisers at an easy but effective level of exertion, we track (and eventually teach them to monitor) their exercise intensities and RPEs along a scale we term the

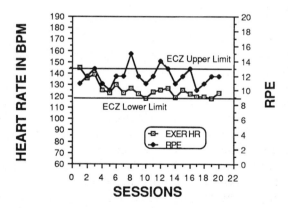

FIGURE 6–1. Effective Comfort Zone Exercise Graph. This figure depicts exercise heart rate (HR) in beats per minute (BPM) on the left ordinate, and the rating of perceived exertion (RPE) on the right ordinate scale. The Effective Comfort Zone (ECZ) is represented by upper and lower HR (60%–75% maximum) and RPE (9–13) limits, which represent, respectively, recommended levels to produce an aerobic (cardiovascular) training effect, but not considered so intense as to produce negative physical or psychological side effects (e.g., burnout).

effective comfort zone (ECZ). This scale represents an exercise level intense enough to be aerobic, but not so intense that it is aversive, or even uncomfortable. Regular feedback is ensured by plotting, or (better) having exercisers plot their exercise heart rates, to assist exercisers in maintaining between 60% and 75% maximum HR (220 − age = max HR). Figure 6–1 illustrates one of these graphs.

Name_____

Date: __   __   __   __   __   __   __
          Sun Mon Tues Wed Thu Fri Sat Average/day

Exercise
      Type_____
      Time_____
      Distance_____

Heart Rate
Before exercise_____
During exercise_____
After exercise_____

Enjoyment Rating
  1. Very unenjoyable   1   1   1   1   1   1   1   1
  2. Unenjoyable   2   2   2   2   2   2   2   2
  3. Neutral   3   3   3   3   3   3   3   3
  4. Enjoyable   4   4   4   4   4   4   4   4
  5. Very enjoyable   5   5   5   5   5   5   5   5

Rating of Perceived
Exertion (RPE)
    (6-20)   _____

Exercised:
  Where   _____

  With whom _____

Comments (number
    and list (#) below)

    _____   _____

Comments (#):

FIGURE 6–2. Exercise Self-Monitoring Form. An illustration of the home and laboratory exercise-monitoring form used in both the treatment and maintenance components of our exercise programs for hypertensives and others. Patients are required to fill this out daily and bring or mail it to therapists on a regular basis.

To enhance the reinforcement during the potentially aversive beginning exercise sessions, we also provide music, group exercise and a considerable amount of praise and positive encouragement from therapists and assistants during as well as after each session. If either the subjective-exertion or enjoyment scale deviates from comfortable/ enjoyable zone for more than two consecutive sessions, we discuss this with the patient and modify the exercise prescription (e.g., reduce intensity) and the laboratory and/or home-exercise reinforcement immediately. We also require patients to monitor exercise at home throughout, beginning with home sessions after the first 2 weeks in the laboratory, so as to enhance generalization to the environment in which they would need to maintain the habit (rather than abruptly switching from lab to home sessions when "graduating" the patient). Our home self-monitoring form is shown in Figure 6–2.

Anecdotally, we are actually discovering a number of hypertensives who were previously noncompliant with their presumably less complex pharmacological regimen who, following this type of behavioral training in shaping and maintaining the exercise habit, adhere quite well to the relatively complex exercise program. This may be due in part to the positive side effects of the exercise (when implemented properly) in combination with the patients' frequently stated desire to do whatever necessary to minimize drug side effects as well as their "sick-role" dependence on medication.

THE EXERCISE PROGRAM

The following portion of the chapter will present the exercise-program format we have come to use for our hypertensives, including the initial screening, exercise/fitness assessments, the exercise-training program itself, and maintenance/follow-up strategies.

Exercise Screening

Given the potential for some forms and intensities of exercise to adversely affect blood pressure and the cardiovascular system, all hypertensives should be medically screened by a physician or exercise physiologist before embarking on any exercise treatment program. Because of the heightened potential for end-organ damage due to the HBP and CHD, all hypertensives should be cleared through a physician, preferably after taking a maximal graded exercise test, before being allowed to exercise in any vigorous fashion. The necessity for this procedure can be explained to the hypertensive in the following manner:

> "Because your high blood pressure puts you at increased risk for coronary heart disease, and damage to your blood vessels, heart and kidneys while also increasing your risk of stroke, it is important that we clear you medically for this exercise program. In that way we can pick up any potential problems that could arise from exercising as well as come up with a much better idea of where to start your exercise program. Finally, this will give us a good baseline to compare your fitness improvements later on. It's not painful, though it may get you pretty tired."

Exercise Testing

The decision about performing a complete physical and/or graded exercise/fitness test rightfully belongs to the physician. Nonetheless, it is incumbent upon the nonphysician exercise program prescriber/provider to conduct some type of screening of any nonmedical (i.e., suspected but not confirmed HBP) as well as medical patients to ensure the patients' safety, and physician consultation is strongly recommended prior to initiation of any strenuous exercising or fitness testing. Exercise physiologists are available on the staffs of many cardiac rehabilitation programs and these professionals can be quite helpful in the screening, assessment, prescription and implementation of safe exercise/fitness programs for patients at a variety of risk levels. If you plan to work with many exercise patients, setting up a consulting relationship with such an expert could be most beneficial. Importantly, they might also be a valuable source of referrals for hypertensive and other patients who are in need of psychological or behavioral interventions. The American College of Sports Medicine (ACSM) is an excellent source of information on locating exercise treatment and assessment specialists as well as for training and certification in exercise testing and prescription (contact ACSM, P.O. Box 1440, Indianapolis, IN 46206; ph. 317-637-9200).

Exercise/Fitness Assessment

Baseline exercise capacity or fitness level should be established prior to initiating any exercise program. Thereafter, regular progress or maintenance checks should be conducted in order to document fitness improvements and to serve as an adherence incentive. Additionally, it is recommended that other dependent variables targeted for change be obtained, such as weight/body fat/girth measures, mood or anxiety levels, as well as measures of baseline fitness level and activity, such as resting and exercise heart rates and routine physical activity levels. The latter might be obtained using the exercise history questionnaire shown in Chapter 3.

This kind of thoroughness in the initial assessment, when followed by regular assessments during treatment, can also help document changes in health status for the patients who do not experience changes in their primary goal (i.e., blood pressure) as soon as they had hoped. Motivation can be maintained, for example, by being able to notify the patient that resting and active heart rates (HR) have significantly decreased, even though their blood pressure has not yet changed during an initial stage of exercise. In our experience and that of others, blood pressure should decrease by the tenth week, though for many this will occur by weeks 6–8.

This comprehensive type of assessment and feedback appears to be extremely important to the majority of individuals undergoing exercise. Moreover, the failure to show any type of change after a reasonable time can cue the program provider to several possibilities: 1) the patient is not adhering well enough to the exercise prescription to produce the desired change, 2) the exercise prescription itself is faulty or inadequate, or 3) the measures are not sensitive enough to assess changes, and perhaps should be altered, supplemented or replaced.

The Graded Exercise ("Stress") Test

There are a number of very safe, well–validated maximal and submaximal exercise tests (Katch, McArdle & McArdle, 1981; ACSM, 1980; Thompson & Martin, 1984). Basically, the maximal tests exercise the individuals to their physical capacity, or exhaustion, or until symptoms appear (i.e., severe shortness of breath, dizziness, leg cramps, ECG abnormalities, chest pain). The submaximal tests stop at a predetermined criterion such as a particular number of minutes or a certain heart rate (e.g., 85% of maximum HR). The maximal test requires the presence of a physician or exercise physiologist, but provides much more complete information as to potential cardiac problems, end-organ damage, etc., and therefore is recommended by most cardiologists for hypertensive patients considering embarking on an exercise program. The maximal graded exercise test has been found extremely safe even for cardiac patients, and is probably the best method of screening hypertensives for potential stress-related problems and for establishing maximal capacity from which to base the exercise prescription.

As with the dietary measure of urine sodium, we recommend that nonphysicians arrange for regular graded exercise testing of their hypertensive patients with experienced medical professionals or exercise physiologists. In our program, we required initial and post-program maximal graded exercise tests for all our participants. These were performed by cardiologists at the medical center in which the project took place. We only admitted hypertensives into our program who had been cleared by their private physician (if any), and we received written clearance from our cardiologist, attesting to the fact that the hypertensives had no observable heart disease or cardiovascular end-organ damage (e.g., kidney dysfunction). Those who were found to have abnormalities were referred back for medical management or were offered other behavioral interventions (e.g., diet, weight reduction, relaxation, smoking treatment) as an adjunct to pharmacologic therapy. Then and only then did we initiate exercise in our hypertensives in sessions at the hospital. Patients were supervised by psychologists and research technicians trained in proper exercise assessment and training procedures, and only moderate levels of exertion (below 85% of their maximum HR) were permitted.

In conjunction with our medical staff, we employed a second, submaximal exercise test ourselves on a monthly basis, in order to document fitness changes and serve as an indirect check on home program adherence. Again, we recommend referral to or collaboration with medical or exercise physiology professionals for all exercise/fitness testing, and employing submaximal or maximal tests of their choosing. Figure 6–3 illustrates monthly progress in fitness in one patient as evidenced by decreasing heart rates to 5-minute bouts of graded exercise work-loads (set at 1/3, 1/2, and 2/3 of initial capacity) and at pre- and

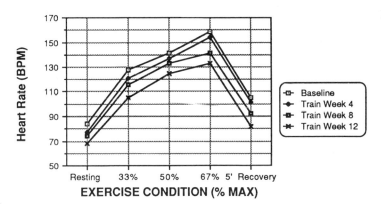

FIGURE 6–3. Graded Fitness/Adherence Test. This figure illustrates a progressive decline in HR levels in BPM across four submaximal exercise tests one month apart. Heart rates are taken at the end of 5 minute periods of rest (sitting), after exercising at standard workloads representing 1/3, 1/2 and 2/3 of their aerobic capacity (determined from initial testing), and 5 minute recovery (sitting). Patients who are exercising regularly (3 times per week or more) would be expected to show decreased HR across time as illustrated here.

post-test rest periods. Generally, the patients found this feedback very motivational, and looked forward to each testing as an opportunity to demonstrate further fitness gains.

The Exercise Prescription

In any exercise prescription, four parameters must be specified: mode, frequency, intensity and duration. The most critical of these is the mode, or type of exercise. Perhaps the most commonly prescribed *mode* or form of noncompetitive exercise is *aerobic exercise*, which has also been termed cardiovascular or endurance exercise, since it primarily improves cardiovascular fitness and work endurance. The research reviewed in this chapter indicates that to effectively lower blood pressure, the exercise should be aerobic. Aerobic exercise refers to repetitive isorythmic activities such as brisk walking, jogging, cycling and swimming—activities which involve the major muscle groups (e.g., legs) in which energy is derived from metabolic processes using a constant flow of oxygen (Cooper, 1968; McArdle et al., 1981). We used bicycle ergometers (more expensive and sturdier stationary cycles with calculated work-resistance settings) and two motorized treadmills in our lab for conducting aerobic exercise.

In order to achieve cardiovascular benefit, these aerobic activities should occur at a minimum *intensity* of 60% to 65% of maximum heart rate, for a *duration* of 15 to 30 minutes or more, and at a minimum *frequency* of three times per week (ACSM, 1978; 1980). Readers interested in more detailed discussions regarding the physiology of exercise are referred to McArdle, Katch and Katch (1981) and Montoye (1978).

As for *duration* of exercise, 30 minutes is an excellent target. This is a sufficient amount of time to produce clinical reductions in blood pressure as well as weight, but is not associated with injury, poor adherence and drop-out (as is 45 minutes, which seems to be too much for the beginning exerciser). Further, this is an easy and convenient block of time which when performed daily (as some will progress to) allows for the amount of physical activity necessary to produce a significant reduction in cardiovascular mortality and morbidity (i.e., 2000 Kcal, or about 3 and 1/2 hours of vigorous exercise per week; Paffenbarger et al., 1985).

With respect to *frequency*, the ACSM guidelines (1980) recommend 3 to 4 times per week for optimal benefits. Actually, for general cardiovascular conditioning, 4 times per week is about as good as 5–7 sessions per week. In fact, the marginal utility of these added sessions is minimum, unless the desire for overall reductions in coronary mortality outweighs the increased risk for injury and drop-out. In our program, we have found that even exercising 3 times per week is sufficient to produce reductions in blood pressure, while constituting a regimen to which patients are able easily to adhere. Though we prescribe 4 sessions per week, we settle for 3 (in fact, we insist on 3, since 2 sessions appear insufficient to produce, or possibly even maintain, the effect).

To establish the exercise *intensity* limits for each hypertensive, we estimate their maximum HR prior to the first exercise session, either from the results of the maximal exercise test (the ending HR), or from a standard formula: 220 − age = Max HR. We then calculate a target, exercise–HR of 70% of this maximum, allowing exercise HRs to range between 60% and 80% of maximum (although we strongly advise keeping the exercise intensity below 75% for the first month or two to maximize enjoyment and minimize the potential for injury and "burn out"). Table 6–5 provides a prescription based on this formula.

Table 6-5. Exercise Prescription Form

Client Name: _____   Date: _____

Physical Data: Age _____   Weight _____ lbs.   Height _____

                 Resting HR _____   BP _____   Body fat _____%

Exercise Mode (circle one):

Walking   Stationary Bicycling   Calisthenics   Swimming

Jogging   Road Bicycling   Aerobic Dance Other: _____

Exercise Frequency: _____ times per week, once each of the following indicated days—

   Su   M   Tu   W   Th   F   Sa

Duration: 2–5 min warm-up

              ___ min exercise

              2–5 min cool-down

Total: ___ min.

Exercise Intensity:

   220 − ____ = _____ × .60 = _____
         Age   100% Heart Rate   Min Exer Heart Rate

                              × .70 = _____
                                      Target Exer Heart Rate

                              × .85 = _____
                                      Max Exer Heart Rate

Technically, the intensity of exercise is calculated in terms of METs, or metabolic equivalent units of energy required to sustain the activity. For example, one MET is equal to 3.5 ml/kg/min of oxygen consumption (i.e., sleeping = 1 MET). Frequently, exercise evaluations and prescriptions are expressed in terms of METS, particularly for cardiac and other patients. Readers are referred to the ACSM book, *Guidelines for graded exercise testing and exercise prescription* (1980) for further information on this.

It should be noted that this formula for recommended training levels, based on estimated maximum HR levels (i.e., 70% max HR), will not be appropriate for patients taking *cardiac inhibitor drugs* such as beta blockers (e.g., Inderal). This is because the drug-mediated suppression of heart rate across all exercise intensities may render the formula-calculated maximum HR unachievable, and therefore invalid. The solution to this invalidation of the formula lies in the essential medical practice of directly testing maximum work capacity in these patients by a physician or exercise physiologist. Medicated patients, generally hypertensives and cardiac patients, should all have undergone a thorough medical workup, including maximal graded exercise testing, while on their cardiac drugs. The maximum HR achieved on the exercise test should then be used, and 70% of that level be targeted as the optimal exercise HR. Additionally, the RPE can be an excellent adjunct in determining appropriate exercise levels. Studies have determined that an RPE of 13 correlates highly with an actual aerobic intensity of 70%. Thus, we instructed our hypertensives who were taking beta blockers to regulate their effort during the exercise by increasing or decreasing the workload setting or speed when pedaling (the bicycle ergometer) or walking such that their exercise perception rating (RPE) approximated "13" (i.e., it feels "somewhat hard").

An important consideration is whether these drugs prevent sufficient cardiovascular involvement needed to produce a training effect. While the studies have been somewhat mixed, the consensus seems to indicate that beta blockers do not prevent the cardiovascular training effect, although the effect may occur more slowly than if the hypertensives were not medicated. Several recent studies (e.g., Pratt et al., 1981) have indicated that these patients may achieve as significant an improvement in cardiovascular fitness as nonmedicated individuals (i.e., up to 30% or more in 10–12 weeks). In any event, all cardiac patients and medicated hypertensives should be carefully supervised by trained medical professionals during all exercise assessment and early training sessions.

EXERCISE SESSIONS

Overview

Similar to the diet modification program described in Chapter 7, the exercise program is divided into four phases, including (a) gradual shaping of the exercise *habit*, (b) lowering blood pressure through increasing levels of aerobic exercise, (c) maintenance of blood pressure lowering through continued exercise in the home, and (d) follow-up contact/testing.

Phase I: Shaping the Exercise Habit

Week 1.

Shaping The Exercise Habit. Our primary emphasis in the first 3 to 4 weeks of exercise training is on effective shaping of the exercise habit. We stress three aspects of an effective exercise program: (1) Comfort; (2) Enjoyability; and (3) Regularity. We spend time debunking some common myths, such as the coaches rule of "No Pain, No Gain." For example, we teach that pain-free, low levels of aerobic exercise are essentially equivalent in their overall cardiovascular training effects to very high levels and, second, if the regimen is more intense and painful, especially during the early stages of training, then the chance of injury and dropout increase precipitously, thereby negating any benefit of all the past improvements in health due to the exercise. We tell patients that, unfortunately, the body "detrains," or loses fitness, even more quickly than it trains, and therefore it is vital to first establish a solid root system for the habit of exercising that can withstand the winds of injuries, loss of exercise partners, moving and travel, sickness, seasonal/weather variations, etc., which so frequently lead to exercise adherence slips, relapses and program dropout.

To "order the steps" of the early exerciser on the path of good adherence, we employ several tools which provide feedback to both the health professional and the exerciser regarding appropriate intensity and enjoyment levels for the exercise. We ask hypertensives to track and self-monitor resting and exercise HRs, as well as exercise RPE and enjoyment levels. We also teach them how to monitor their breathing, so as to keep exercise intensity at a level where they are not breathless. We stress their ability to talk to one another while exercising without shortness of breath (SOB).

The *warm-up and cool-down* is very important and we spend time in the first session or two on these exercise enhancers and injury preventors. We explain that the function of the warm-up is to shift blood to the muscles to be used (e.g., legs) so no injuries or stiffness will occur as a result of overstretching a cold, tight muscle. We tell them never to stretch a cold muscle due to the chance of tearing or injuring the muscles, but to perform the exercise in a much slower, easier fashion for about 2–5 minutes. The cool-down, similar to the warm-up, allows the body and muscles to gradually slow down, so that blood will not pool, and exertional waste byproducts (e.g., blood lactate) can be carried away rather than deposited in the muscles, thereby causing stiffness and discomfort later. We ask patients to practice this, monitoring their performance closely until they are adhering to the instructions comfortably. Regarding *stretching*, we generally recommend against it, since many of the injuries in our community exercise program were due to improper stretching (e.g., bouncing, "making it burn") of cold and tight muscles. We instructed patients that if they must stretch, to wait until they are well warmed-up, preferably toward the end, or following the exercise.

Tracking blood pressure is, of course, a key feature in our laboratory-based exercise sessions; however, we suggest that blood pressure be taken only once a week, during rest (at least 5 minutes sitting) and before the exercise session. For home-based programs the patients themselves can take their blood pressure. Therapists are well-advised to supplement this with periodic clinic blood pressure determinations.

The first week of exercise should be used to acquaint the patient with the program philosophy (exercise can and should be enjoyable and easy) and procedures to gradually shape the exercise habit, *and* to ensure that their first session is painless, easy and fun (or, at worst, not unenjoyable). To help ensure that subsequent sessions in the early program are easily manageable and less potentially problematic, we prescribe at least one day of rest in between exercise sessions. In this way, exercise sessions never occur on consecutive days unless a makeup session is required.

Because our fitness interventions have occurred in a medical facility with all the appropriate exercise/fitness assessment and training equipment and personnel, we felt it was an advantage to include a greater percentage of laboratory sessions—where patients could be closely supervised and shaped by our staff—in the early stages of the program. We understand that a majority of the readers may not have this advantage. Thus, we are providing an outline to a program that can easily be adapted to the home setting almost exclusively. We do caution the health care professional to insert as many clinic or lab sessions as possible (at least once a week, even if briefly) in the beginning. In the

Table 6-6. Schedule of Sessions

Setting	Week													
	1	2	3	4	5	6	7	8	9	10	11	12	13	14
# Clinic Sessions	2	2	2	2	2	1	1	1	1	1	0	1	0	1
# Home Sessions	0	1	2	2	2	3	3	3	3	3	4	3	4	3

event that the reader refers the patient to an ongoing exercise program, we recommend that the therapist attend at least some sessions to get a better idea of the program, particularly with respect to the overall learning environment, and the training/shaping methods.

At first, we require patients to come twice per week during the first month. This is followed by two home (and two program/clinic) sessions the third week. Thus, by the end of week 3, all participants have been shaped up to the optimal exercise frequency of 4 times per week. The advantages of this early home intervention are as follows: (1) Even if exercisers miss one home session (which often occurs, especially early on), they have still met the aerobic criterion of 3 times per week; (b) less program personnel time is required; and (c) early home sessions help to more completely establish the exercise habit in the home environment, thereby maximizing stimulus (setting) generalization, and increasing the probability of long-term maintenance of the exercise regimen once treatment proper has been completed. Table 6–6 shows this schedule of sessions across 12 treatment weeks and two maintenance sessions.

Table 6–7 provides a general session-by-session Exercise Sessions Format. Key features of our recommended 12-week (plus maintenance/fading sessions) exercise program include the gradual shaping up of frequency of sessions in the clinic and at home, and, at week 5, the initiating of fading of clinic sessions (in adherent hypertensives), while at the same time increasing home sessions from 2 to 3. The content of each week and each session are presented and summarized both in the table and in the following section.

Our *initial exercise instructions* to the hypertensive are as follows:
You have now been cleared for exercise, and we are ready to begin. As you know, we believe that this exercise program will very likely lower your blood pressure. Similar regimens have lowered the pressures of many others like you. You may even be able to reduce or eliminate your blood pressure medication (or, for those already faded off their medications: not have to go back on your medications), but that will depend on how quickly and how well your particular cardiovascular system responds to the exercise and on how dependable you are in following the program.
We are about to teach you a whole new way of exercising that we think you will enjoy. Forget that you may have been told "no pain, no gain"—that for exercise to really work it has to hurt. This is absolutely

Table 6-7. Exercise Sessions Format for 12-Week+ Program

Week	Session	Content
		Phase I: Shaping of Exercise Habit
1	1	*Introduction, rationale & myth smashing.* Explain and fit Heartrate (HR) monitor, warm-up and cool-down. Conduct 5–15 min exercise on stationary bicycle (B) or treadmill (T) or other @ 50–65% max Heartrate; 10–12 RPE 4–5 Enjoyability and no breathlessness. Sign Contract.
	2	Exercise Session similar to previous session @ same RPE and Enjoyment as Session I. Discuss Feedback effects on exer adherence & performance
2	3	10–15 min exer session with 2 min rest, then 5–10 min @ 60–70% maximum heartrate; RPE < 13; Enjoyment > 3. Client begins recording own data. Discuss Reinforcement.
	4	Same Exercise as Session 3 Assign home session Give HR monitor & home-monitoring forms Discuss Social Support
3	5	Review home session Exercise Session Begin exerciser adjusting workloads on own Discuss distraction/thoughts
	6	Exercise: Two 15 min sessions Discuss Stimulus Control Assign 2 home sessions
4	7	Check home sessions, problem-solve. Exercise same as previous session. Exerciser conducts session, including load adjustments & recording Begin Discussion of how to handle exercise relapse/slips. Assign 2 home sessions
	8	Check home session & self-monitoring forms Two 15 min exercise periods.
		Phase II: Exercise Increases Until BP Lowered **Begin Home Generalization**
5	9	Exercise session same as previous week. Assign 3 home exercise sessions.
6	10	Review home self-monitoring. Discuss 3 home sessions. Patient conduct own exercise session with minimal supervision similar to previous week. Discuss fading and generalization training (to home setting). Assign 3 home sessions.
7	11	Review home sessions. Problem solve. Exercise session same as previous session.

Table 6-7 (*Continued*)

Week	Session	Content
		Discuss social support, invite family to Clinic to watch and/or exercise.
		Assign 3 home sessions.
8	12	Review home program & problem solve.
		Have patient show family member(s) how to use equipment and exercise.
		Dual exercise session with patient and family member.
		Assign 3 home sessions.
9	13	Review home exercise and problem solve.
		Similar exercise session.
		Patient & family member(s) exercise.
		Provide ample praise to both.
		Discuss importance of praise during exercise, review distraction and thought control.
		Assign 3 home sessions.

	⋗	Phase III: Complete Home Generalization
10	14	Exercise Session with family member(s)
		Review home sessions:
		If session & home adherence ≥ 80%
		Then reduce to 1 Clinic session per 2 weeks.
		Also:
		IF RESTING, DBP < 90 MM HR, CONTINUE SESSIONS FADING; IF NOT, RETURN TO START OF PHASE II (ONLY ONCE).
		Discuss Relapse Prevention.
		Assign 4 home sessions each of next two weeks.
12	15	Review home session monitoring forms
		Problem solve with patient and family member(s):
		*If 80% adherence past 2 weeks, then fade to 3 monthly sessions, then 3 mo. followups.
		*If not, return to weekly session until ≥ 80% adherence.
		Also: If DBP ≥ 90 mm Hg—
		Refer to physician for possible drug therapy, and/or add weight/diet/stress interventions.
		Exercise 30 min, using preferred home exercise
		Discuss Relapse Recovery Strategies.
		Discuss long-term contract for maintenance
14	16	Review home self-monitoring Problem Solving.
		Regular exer session (30 min).
		Discuss relapse prevention.
		Sign Long-term Maintenance and Follow-up Contract.

	Phase IV: Long Term Maintenance and Follow Up
Monthly Follow-up (×3)	Review Records 30 min Exercise session
3-Month Follow-ups (×3)	Review Records 15–30 min exercise session optional.

false. In fact, just the opposite is true. The easier it is, down to a point, the better it is for you, and the more likely you are to stick with it!

Believe it or not, our first goal is to get you in the habit of exercising regularly. If you don't exercise regularly, then no matter how good it is at controlling your blood pressure, it will stop working when you stop exercising. We do this in several ways. First, we make sure the early exercise experiences you have with us are painless, and easy, if not downright enjoyable! If at any time you are uncomfortable, very fatigued or just plain not liking your exercise, please inform me or one of the assistants right away so we can work on adjusting your program to better suit you. This is very important, and is our first rule.

Our second rule has to do with competition. Since we will be having you exercise with others like you, try not to compare yourself and your program with them. Everyone is different and progresses at a different pace. Comparing yourself with others will amost always be frustrating, especially when they may be progressing a bit faster than you. Remember, too, that some start fast and then slow up, while others may start seemingly slow, and then catch a "second wind" and really take off some weeks down the line. In this game, the tortoise *always* beats the hare to the finish . . . in this case becoming fit for life. We want you to be your body's best friend and listen carefully to it so it can tell you when it is ready to push a little harder or when you need to back off a little. Any questions?

Now, to help us know what is the best exercise level for you, we will be using several methods. First is how you feel. There are two ways to get at this. First is the subjective: To tell us how much you are exerting yourself, as you perceive it, we will be asking you to rate your exertional level using this scale (show *RPE* scale, Table 6–3, on exercise room wall and/or self-monitoring form), marking the number down here (show *exercise self-monitoring form*, Figure 6–2). Also, we want to know how you are enjoying your exercise, so sometime in the middle of your exercise session, please note your *enjoyment level* (show scale posted on wall and/or on self-monitoring form, Table 6–4). We will watch to see that you do not have more than one or two sessions in which you fail to get into the enjoyable range. Please remember the rule: If it hurts or the exercise is consistently unenjoyable, then there is something wrong that we need to fix with your program. Now, some days you may be feeling a little down or stressed, but this shouldn't happen consistently or we're not doing our job. We would like you to take responsibility for your exercise program, and here is a way to start—by keeping up with your data and informing us when things are going well, or not so well.

A second means of telling your intensity is more exact—your heart rate. The best measure of your exercise intensity level is usually your heart rate (HR). Remember, they looked at your heart rate during the exercise-stress test. We can too, with either a portable *heart-rate monitor* or by taking a quick pulse (show Exercentry or other HR monitoring device, and have patient put it on, or instruct in taking pulse). At 5-minute intervals in your exercise we would like you to note your pulse reading on the meter or take your wrist (radial) or neck (carotid) pulse with your fingers for 6 seconds adding a zero—and record the HR level on your monitoring form. In this way (particularly with monitoring device with preset alarms) you can get regular feedback in keeping your HR within that we call the *effective* comfort zone (ECZ), of 60% of 75% of your maximum HR (show patient how their maximum was determined from exercise test, or from formula; see Table 6–5). We would like you to exercise such that you keep your HR within these limits (tell them what their 60% and 75% HRs are, and have them write them down on self-monitoring form). (For those with monitor devices: The alarms on this device will help you to stay within these limits because it will beep when you go above or below them, cueing you to speed up or slow down in the exercising you are doing.) At first, we will monitor you closely and help you keep within these comfortable but effective limits, for example by changing the tension/workload on the stationary bicycle for you, or increasing or decreasing the speed of the treadmill or your walking pace. Later, you will be able to do this on your own. Thus, your task will be to keep within the ECZ, and to have a graph of your exercise HRs that looks like this (show Figure 6–1, and explain how they are to keep up graph). Any questions on all this?

Let's start with our first session of exercise, after taking your resting blood pressure and HR for our records. Each day you come to exercise, we would like you to dress (put on your HR monitor), and get your data forms. Then, we'll start you on either the bicycle or treadmill for 15 minutes, then switch you to the other for 15 minutes. (Home programs: Begin your walking/jogging/cycling slowly the way we are about to show you.) For the first week, we'll just start with an easy 10 to 15 minutes on just one of your choice, then we'll add the second 15 minute round by the end of the second week. Let's start you here (bike or treadmill set to workload/speed/elevation reflecting 60% of tested maximum, or to low level and adjusted upward slowly until HR stabilizes between 60% and 75% of maximum) . . . How does that feel? Good.

There is a third way to tell if you are overexerting yourself. That is, you can observe things about your response to the exercise. These include your breathing, which should not be labored—if you are huffing and puffing or unable to have a conversation without gasping for breath, you are going too hard, so ease up—your sweating, and your skin color and temperature. You should not be sweating profusely, unless, of course you are in a hot room or outside when it's very warm. Here in our air-conditioned laboratory you should hardly be sweating at all. Finally, your skin should not become bright red and flushed, or very hot. If it does, you are overworking and need to back off some. We will watch for some of these signs of overexertion, and hope you will too. We'd like for you to become quite good at this kind of monitoring so that for your home sessions, and when you are exercising on your own after the program ends, you will be able to keep pacing yourself properly and avoiding burnout and injury. Any questions on all that?

Why don't we review what you have just learned. Can you tell me how you are to exercise and how to monitor your exercise exertion? Good. Let's do a 10-to-15-minute session now. Very good. . . .

For this first week, we stress the ease and enjoyability of exercising, and pull out all the stops to ensure that their patients' initial experiences reflect this! We carefully supervise every minute of their first few

Table 6-8. Suggested Exercise/Jogging Feedback & Praise

General Positive
(When you can't think of other positive things to lead off with)

+ It's good to see you out here today.
+ Way to reinforce that exercise habit—keep up the good work
+ Your attendance has been good (if it has)—you're well on the way to really making this exercise a habit.
+ Doesn't this beat lying around getting fat and heart disease?
+ You look like you're enjoying this—good for you.
+ I like to see so many people here—thanks for coming.
+ I love to see all these people out here improving their health and enjoying themselves.

Pacing/Intensity

+ Your pace/intensity level looks great/perfect/just right . . . keep it up.
+ Excellent/good pace! . . . nice going.
+ Your breathing sounds just right . . . good level of exercise.
+ I like your exercise level . . . looks like it is pretty comfortable, does it seem that way to you?
+ That's good . . . your pace seems not too fast or slow . . . just right.
+ Does your pace feel as good as it looks?

? Would you say your pace is too fast, too slow or just right?
? How does this (your) pace feel?
? Can you talk comfortably at this pace? That's good/try slowing down a bit.
? Does this pace feel good? It looks/*good/a little too slow/a little too fast/*
? Is this an enjoyable pace or are you finding it a little difficult?

− You seem to be breathing pretty hard, why don't you try slowing down/backing off some.
− You might find it more enjoyable if you'll slow your pace down a bit.
− You seem to be huffing and puffing some . . . try slowing down . . . you'll enjoy it more.
− I can tell you're having trouble talking and jogging/walking/cycling . . . that must mean you're going too fast.
− You may be going a little too slow (what's your HR been?) Why don't you speed up a touch—but not too much.

Form (jogging/walking)

+ Your *posture* is great!
+ Your *back* is straight, good going.
+ I like the way your *back* is straight and your *upper trunk* is relaxed and balanced right above the middle of your hips.
+ Your *neck and shoulders* look good—nice and level and relaxed.
+ Your *form* is good/great—keep it up.
+ You run/walk very *efficiently*—you look great.
+ You're really improving on your *form*, for example. . . .
+ Your *arms and hands* are great . . . way to keep those arms relaxed but not floppy (90% break and close to body, swiveling 2″–6″, just above hips, and your *hands* are nicely cupped but not tight).
+ With good form like that, you must be relaxed and comfortable.
+ Your _____ looks so good, can I tell others to watch or jog with you to pick up that positive habit?
+ Your *foot* (heel) placement looks good.
+ That's the way to relax your *foot and leg* on the recovery.
+ You're *running* very *smoothly*—no bouncing at all. Great!
+ Your hips are nice and loose—that lets you stride smoothly.

Table 6-8. *Continued*

- You're bouncing a bit too much—can you tell?—try running more smoothly.
- Straighten your back—almost like you're going to fall over backwards (physically straighten then with hand on shoulder and back). You'll find it much more comfortable, tho' a bit awkward at first.

General Health
+ You're looking more trim—have you lost some weight too?
+ Your HR's been good—right on target.
+ I've noticed your BP's come down some. That's great!

? How's your resting/post-run HR? Are you in the aerobic range?
? Are you finding any positive physical changes yet?
? Your resting HR is somewhat higher: Have you changed your diet, exercise or work habits? Losing sleep? Higher stress?

- Your HR suggests you're going a bit too fast. Try slowing down some—your body will thank you.
- Your resting HR appears higher. Try slowing down more, in general. You might also want to cut down on stimulants such as nicotine, caffeine, etc., get more sleep if that's a problem or try to cut down on stress (i.e., —back off some at work—take more breaks).

---

sessions, giving ample praise and feedback to the patients for the first 2 to 4 weeks, and recommend whenever possible that even home-based programs begin with supervised exercise training. This early training might include live or videotape modeling and careful debriefing and data analysis, especially for those who will be exercising on their own or in less supervised settings. For organized programs, we recommend choosing or providing a program with a good staff-to-client ratio (for example, *not* a large aerobics dance class, at first). Our staff-to-patient ratio is generally 1:2, and sometimes up to 1:4. Ideally, we do not recommend having more than four patients per staff person, and no more than two patients per staff person during early sessions (when individual sessions are best). We subsequently integrate patients into groups with less individualized staff attention after about the second or third week; we allow (even encourage) more independence as patients demonstrate their ability to stay within the recommended HR, RPE, enjoyability and workload limits, and are able to operate the equipment (i.e., BP cuff, treadmill controls, HR monitors). We find that it is particularly important to provide ample praise during the exercise, especially because it appears to have a more powerful impact on adherence and enjoyability then. Some sample praise and feedback statements and comments are contained in Table 6–8.

Especially early in the training, we always scrutinize the RPE and enjoyability ratings of the patients. Generally we take RPE only once in the middle of the exercise bout, although in the first couple of sessions, we may request these ratings about every 5 minutes or at any workload-transition point. We also carefully monitor visible signs of overexertion (we are rarely concerned about underexertion, especially during the first several weeks of Phase I), such as heavy breathing or sweating, turning red, frowning during exercise or significant muscle tension. Perhaps one of the most important features of the first phase of the exercise program is the signing and agreeing to the terms of the behavioral contract. This contract, shown in Figure 6–4, makes use of significant others (preferably family members) from the patient's home environment to help track and consequate exercise adherence and nonadherence. We do not assign home exercise sessions until the end of the second full exercise week, to give patients at least four model sessions on which to base their home exercise. This also gives us ample time to problem solve any impediments to a successful session in the home environment, and to rehearse with the patients exactly what we would like them to do. We have found that the risk of having patients exercising on their own too soon (we refer here more to the adherence-burnout risk rather than health risk), is more than outweighed by the advantage of very early, and thus more comprehensive, generalization training to the environment in which they will ultimately need to maintain their exercise program. Our approach is somewhat unique in this way; however, our adherence results are so encouraging that we have made this a core training component.

The measures we obtain during the first week are obtained throughout treatment and follow-up. *Resting blood pressure* is the primary measure for assessing improvements and treatment efficacy. We take great care in BP assessment and in training staff in blood pressure measurement (see Chapter 3). We recommend that resting blood pressure be taken approximately once a week under systematic conditions (take twice following a 5-to-10-minute rest period with patient sitting comfortably in a quiet room, with at least 1 minute in between measures, and recording the second blood pressure or the average between the two). For the resting BP we generally recommend using a mercury column sphygmomanometer, which is likely to be more accurate and doesn't need calibration as do the aneroid-type monitors. Automated BP devices can also be highly accurate; however, any movement whatsoever can invalidate the readings. During early sessions (especially the first week or two), we also obtain *resting HR* (after sitting 5 to 10 minutes), and *exercise HR* about every 5 minutes using portable HR monitors, or 6-second radial or carotid pulse sample ($\times$ 10 to calculate beats per minute). Rating of perceived exertion (RPE) and enjoyability ratings are also obtained and recorded up to every 5 minutes during exercise.

EXERCISE/HEALTH CONTRACT

I, _____agree to:

    (a) exercise:

        _____ times per week.

        for _____ min, at a minimum intensity of _____ (HR/RPE/METS)

        and a maximum intensity of _____ (HR/RPE/METS).

    (b) Record the exercise on my weekly self-monitoring form.

    (c) Keep my appointments or call in advance to reschedule:

        (_____, extension _____).

In return, _____agrees to reinforce these
changes in one of the following ways each week when I meet my exercise goals.

    (a) _____

    (b) _____

    (c) _____

2. Spouse or Helper

I,_____agree to the following:

    (a) Health behavior change:_____ _____times per week.

    (b) _____

    (c) _____

In return, I (patient)_____agree to reinforce these
changes in one of the following ways each week when I meet my goals.

    (a) _____

    (b) _____

    (c) _____

3. Effective dates of the contract:_____

4. Signatures: PATIENT_____

           SPOUSE or HELPER_____

           CLINICAL PROFESSIONAL_____

FIGURE 6–4. Exercise/Health Contract. This figure represents a standard contract used in our program, in which the patient and a significant other (usually spouse or other family member) agree to provide reinforcement contingent upon fulfillment of exercise goals. The helper contract for their own health-behavior change shown at the bottom (2) is an optional component we have found is a requested and desirable feature for a number of family members who want to improve their own health at the same time.

We take some blood pressures, including one during and following exercise in the first week (to ensure that BP is not dropping precipitously [i.e., 10 mm Hg diastolic], which might indicate heart problems) using an aneroid (dial-type) sphygmomanometer. We like the aneroid cuffs for postsession measures for several reasons: First, they are easier to operate and handle, and less delicate, an advantage when we train the patients to take their own postsession BP after the second week; and second, we use the kind that show a light and that beep at detection of the Korotkoff sounds. In a noisy exercise lab, this is no small feature. Thirdly, they are generally less expensive (about $50 to $70 as opposed to $100 to $200).

Week 2. The clinician may want at this point to establish laboratory-fitness baseline. We were not qualified to conduct a maximal-graded exercise test, such as was completed by our cardiologist to screen out those with more serious problems; but because of our training in this area (cf., American College of Sports Medicine [ACSM], 1978, 1980) and our well-equipped exercise facility, we employ a simple, repeatable, *submaximal-graded exercise test* (described earlier in this chapter). We don't, of course, recommend this to everyone and will not therefore go into detail at this point. We might recommend, however, that the health care professional consider arranging for monthly submaximal exercise tests to be conducted in some exercise, rehabilitation or medical program, keeping in mind that, strategically, it is unwise to overstress a neophyte, untrained individual with repeated maximal-output tests. Clearly, although we appreciate the desirability of documenting the fitness progress on a regular basis, we also stress the importance of avoiding in the new exerciser early contact with the aversive consequences of high levels of exercise.

In the event the submaximal-graded exercise test is performed, we then note to the hypertensives that they will be given the same test at 5 and 10 weeks and at set follow-up points, for comparison to this baseline test to assess fitness improvement. We explain that as they adhere to the 3-to-4-days per week exercise regimen, then their HR should be lower to the three workloads, and at rest and recovery points, reflecting their improved cardiopulmonary endurance (i.e., they can do more physical work for longer with lower HRs). We always praise participants for their performance and completion of the test, no matter how poor their fitness is. We never discuss with them how their initial performance compares with others, so as not to induce unhealthy competition or to invite negative self-statements for their comparatively poor fitness. We use the tests only for comparison with their own past performances, as a yardstick for progress, and as an indirect measure of home adherence (this is particularly useful for follow-up visits, when patients are in maintenance and not coming in for regular training in the clinic or laboratory). As additional measures of fitness for future comparisons, we obtain weights on patients, and may check skinfolds at the baseline and at 5-week and 10-week testing points.

The second half of the Week 2, Day 1 session or, in the case where no exercise assessment is conducted, the beginning of the session, is a duplicate of the first week's prescription—10 to 15 minutes on the bicycle ergometer—to vary the involved muscles slightly, and for the added benefit of no weight bearing in the second period when they are more tired (for testing on the ergometers, reverse this order). We adjust the workload down slightly from the previous week, since they may be tired from the test. We carefully monitor RPE, enjoyment and visible signs of fatigue or stress, and may even stop them at 5 minutes. In the event that another exercise is to be used, such as brisk walking, we translate workload to speed, and train participants to adjust their exercise intensity to a comfortable level. Again, we are not nearly so concerned with reaching the aerobic minimum of 20 minutes as we are with making sure the exercise is easy and enjoyable.

The second exercise day in Week 2 is similar: Two 10-to-15-minute exercise bouts are conducted in the fashion suggested for Week 1, alternating the treadmill and bicycle ergometer (note that the equipment is not necessary for training, because patients can walk/jog briskly around the program grounds, for example, but it does allow for observation within a single room, variety in exercise, and is considered novel and motivating, if not somewhat fun to operate, by many patients in our experience). At this point we begin to encourage patients to start recording their own data, including resting/exercise HRs, RPE, and enjoyment. We progressively shape patients to eventually record all their measures, including postexercise BP, so that by about the middle of the 12-week treatment program they are able to accurately measure and record, for example, HRs, RPE, enjoyment, time exercising, workloads, and BP. That allows the program therapists and assistants to spend more time on providing feedback and praise, and problem solving.

The important role of praise and other forms of *reinforcement* for exercising are stressed with the patients. We discuss what they like to do, and have commented on, and problem-solve ways for this to be made contingent on exercising. We especially focus on the effectiveness of praise and social distraction during the exercise itself, and model this for them whenever they are exercising with us (we try to average a positive comment about their exercise, attendance, improving appearance and fitness, pacing, etc., about once every 2 minutes—more often the first week or two, fading to around once in each 15-minute exercise bout toward the latter end of treatment). We also encourage them to ask for praise and encouragement from family members for their exercising.

Thus, usually by the end of the second week and possibly by the third in more unfit individuals, the exercise session consists of: (a) changing to exercise clothes (for blood-pressure assessment days: sitting for 10 minutes with no talking, e.g., reading and having staff member take their resting BP twice); (b) putting on HR monitor; (c) 2 to 5 minutes easy warm-up exercise at very low intensity (note here that we do not encourage any stretching of cold muscles prior to exercise, but rather an initial very gradual warm-up to shunt blood to the muscles to be used); (d) exercising at low aerobic intensity (60% to 70% maximum HR; RPE = 10–12) on treadmill, walking course, or bicycle ergometer for 15 minutes; (e) recording RPE and enjoyment level every 5 minutes; (f) a brief rest of 1 to 2 minutes, walking and easy stretching; (g) exercising for another 15 minutes on alternative equipment or activity (walk course, treadmill, or ergometer, whichever not used in the first period); (h) recording RPEs and enjoyment levels at 5 minute intervals again; and (i) walking or cycling easily for 2 to 5 minutes as cool-down, with perhaps some very gentle stretching to loosen up any stiff muscles.

A final component in the second session of week two consists of the assignment of the first *home exercise session*. We pass out the exercise-monitoring form (Figure 6–3) and instruct patients on how, when and where to exercise. It is convenient, time efficient and even helpful (i.e., it induces distraction from discomfort of exercise) to discuss these things during the latter 15-minute exercise period, or when they are more stationary on the ergometer—a time when we would find ourselves providing many of our instructions to patients. At the end of the second week, patients were instructed to begin doing one extra exercise session per week on their own, either at or near home or work. The requirements were that it be similar with respect to the type of exercise (walking, jogging or stationary cycling), overall intensity (i.e., max HR, RPE), and duration (minimum 15 minutes, maximum 30 minutes), and, whenever possible, on the day after a nonexercise day (we asked them to avoid exercising two days in a row at first, to allow full recovery from any initial stiffness, fatigue, etc.). We then issued them one of the HR monitors to help keep their intensity within the 60% to 75% maximum HR limits we used in the lab, and briefly discussed when, where and with whom it might be best to exercise.

Week 3. After assessing their resting BP, we first review the clients' home exercise self-monitoring, something we do regularly each new week. If there are problems, we discuss solutions and alternatives until an acceptable one is arrived at and an attack plan made. Then we conduct two exercise periods of 15 minutes (the latter could be 10 to 15 minutes, depending on fatigue factors, etc.). During the session, we discuss the importance of *distracting thoughts* during exercise, and how they could insulate them from the common discomforts and boredom of exercise (especially a stationary activity such as bicycle ergometry work). Our instructions were as follows:

> The results of studies on exercise motivation indicate that what a person thinks about during exercise can have a profound effect on how they do, and more importantly, how long they stick with their exercise program. Generally, the more you think about the exercise, your body and how it feels, the more you will tune into the routine discomforts that accompany exercising, and the less enjoyable it will be for you. One study, in fact (our own), showed that people who could be taught to do the opposite—think distracting, anything-but-exercise thoughts—were much more likely to stay with their exercise program over the short and the longer run! It makes sense. There are some discomforts with taking a body and heart and lungs that have, for a number of reasons, become very out of shape to a much more highly fit state. It can also be quite boring at times, especially if you are stationary, with no change in scenery such as on our bicycles. Well, there's a cure for that—distract yourself when you are exercising: Read, talk, listen to music, watch TV, let your mind drift, but try not to think about the exercise and how it feels. There are two exceptions to this rule.
>
> First, if you experience an important pain that you cannot ignore, such as extreme fatigue, chest pain, or a leg cramp, you must pay attention and take corrective action—for example, by lowering your workload or the speed you are exercising, or by stopping.
>
> Second, when your body and heart and lungs get to the point of fitness that the signals from your body are *pleasant*, then by all means attend and enjoy! This may not happen for some weeks or months, so don't worry if it doesn't. It took you a long time to get out of shape, so please understand that you will need a little time to become fit.
>
> One of the best ways to distract is to talk with others, especially those you like. You may have noticed that we talk to patients quite a lot when they are exercising. This is no coincidence. We do it because we know it helps you enjoy the exercise more. And, after all, that is our primary goal these first few weeks. To help you have pleasant distractions in our laboratory, from now on we will have music during the exercise sessions, and we would like you to bring in your favorite music tape, or suggest to us your favorites, and we will try to provide them for you. In addition, bring in any reading material that you would enjoy reading. For your home sessions we recommend that you exercise with a Walk man-type radio, or with a family member or friend, or that you use other methods of distraction that we have suggested or use here. Picking a place to exercise that has many distractions, such as a park, zoo, athletic field with many activities, a shopping mall, or even a busy

city sidewalk, can also help to provide the physical environment for enjoyable thought-wandering. We'll help you learn how to do this, and it should really pay dividends in enhancing your exercise motivation, or at least minimizing your discomfort, so try it, we really think you'll like it!

By the second exercise session of Week 3 we encourage patients to try the full two 15-minute exercise periods, with about a 2-minute rest period in between, if they have not already achieved that level—though most are already at that level by the end of the second week. Individuals who desire to do more we generally encourage to hold off and follow the simple program rather than pushing it to the point of discomfort.

As in Week 2, we assign a home exercise session (and issue a HR monitoring device) before the patient leaves that day; however, we add a second home session at this point. Thus, they are asked to exercise twice in the lab with us each week and twice at home during that week. This is important for two reasons: First, in the event patients miss one of their two home sessions, or if they miss a lab session, they can still meet the aerobic criterion of 3 times per week (which will occur about half the time). It's a cushion of sorts, but a very valuable one in a limited-time exercise program (our medical consultants told us, "You have 3 months to lower their BP with exercise . . . otherwise back on meds!"). Second, as noted earlier, it initiates generalization to the home environment early so as to enhance the probability that the exercise will be maintained once the formal program sessions are faded and then discontinued.

Week 4. The format for the fourth exercise program week is very similar to the third week, except that the patients are shaped to take on more of the session measures and recording responsibilities on their own. In particular, they should be taking their own postexercise BP by now, and setting and adjusting their HR monitors and workloads on the treadmill and bicycle ergometer. Also, a new topic—stimulus-control techniques—is presented.

Our instructions regarding the understanding and use of *stimulus control* are consistent with the following:

> Today we are going to teach you about how to use special cues and prompts to help you want to exercise as well as actually exercise, and how to avoid those that influence you in the opposite direction. We know that things in our environment—events, places, cues, even the clothes you wear—can greatly influence behaviors such as exercising. Remember, we talked about how important convenience is to participation in exercise. For example, if you have to drive a long way to pick up your exercise clothes, then drive to the exercise facility, most people would be unlikely to keep this up for very long. An option would be to always carry your exercise clothing in the car with you, and

choose an exercise program that is convenient and easy. It is more likely that you would then exercise more regularly, especially if there are many cues in your home and work places for exercising.

What cues you expose yourself to can really influence whether you exercise. You can make this work for you by filling your home and work environment with many reminders to exercise. For example, try to keep your exercise clothes handy and visible; hang around fitness-oriented people and/or your exercise facility: don't get involved in other activities close to your normal exercise time; encourage your exercising friends to call you to go exercise; wear an exercise watch; prominently display on a table or a chart your exercise-program attendance and fitness improvements, and so on. Another very important way to cue yourself to exercise is to show up at your appointed exercise facility on time, no matter how you feel. Our motto is, show up, dress to exercise, and at least start. You don't have to do much if you don't feel well, but often when you bring the body, the mind and feelings follow. The best cue to exercise sometimes is to just show up. Then, upon seeing the other exercisers, the equipment, the therapists, and all the individuals encouraging you, you are much more likely to exercise.

Conversely, you are much less likely to exercise if you are at home, in your nice comfy recliner in front of the TV. Don't get into that situation. Go and exercise first. Then do those enjoyable things. The only excuses for not coming are: fever; significant injury or illness; hospitalization; or a personal, work, or family emergency. You can help motivate yourself to exercise by effective use of the cues (and reinforcement, too) available to you in your environment. Now, let's talk about how we can harness those from your particular living situation to work with the reinforcement you are already using to give you the habit of exercising.

Week 5. The fifth week is the optional fitness-test week, in which programs may wish to arrange to have a second submaximal-graded exercise test conducted. Otherwise, a full session of regular exercise should be provided, and determinations as to whether the patient should be advanced to more home sessions (and correspondingly fewer clinic sessions) should just be based on attendance, and possibly blood-pressure response to the exercise.

The fitness test is used, when feasible, to assess fitness improvements more objectively, and to provide an indirect check on home-exercise adherence as well as feedback to the patient. A comparison is then made between HRs achieved in the two tests (shown in Figure 6–3). Also, the exercise-adherence levels are calculated for the previous 4 weeks, home-adherence and treatment-satisfaction checks are conducted (Tables 6–9 and 6–10), and a decision is made as to whether to institute the session fading of Phase II (transfering from program to home sessions).

To advance to the second phase, the following should be present: (a) At least one current-test exercise HR or recovery HR should be below

Table 6-9. Home Collateral Check

Client/Patient's Name _____

Date _____

Informant's Name _____   Relationship _____

                                                                        phone # _____

Phone Interview for Exercise Adherence

1. Is your husband/wife/(   ) still exercising?

2. What kinds of exercise has he/she been doing the past month and how often?

3. Does he/she have good weeks and bad weeks, or is he pretty consistent from week to week?

4. Has he/she ever missed exercising for more than a few days in a row? If yes, describe when and what were the circumstances if known.

5. How many minutes does he/she spend exercising each time?

6. Have you ever noticed him/her taking his heart rate while exercising? Before exercising? After exercising?

7. Does (   ) ever exercise with anyone?

8. (If informant cannot give much information, e.g., if exercise not done at home)—Is there anyone else we could call to ask about (   )'s exercise program?

the baseline measure (usually all will be); and/or (b) the exercise attendance and home adherence should be 80% or above (this is an arbitrary figure, but the decision should reflect that individuals have exercised at the aerobic threshold of 3 times per week for at least 3 of the 4 weeks, and demonstrated that they could effectively complete home exercising). In addition, resting BP is taken (before testing), as well as weight and body fat measures. In most individuals, BP should be decreasing by now, but this is not essential. A number of our hypertensives did not show a significant decline in BP until the sixth or eighth week, with a few taking a full 10 weeks to normalize or exhibit clinically significant reductions in BP (i.e., ≥ 5 mm Hg).

If the individuals meet the above criteria, and most should, then they can be progressed to the Phase II of blood-pressure lowering, and beginning home generalization. If not, then we recommend one of three options: (1) they can be continued in Phase I for 4 more weeks, or until the advance criteria are met; (2) they could be placed in weight/diet or stress-management programs if this has not already been attempted; or (3) they could be referred back to their physician for drug therapy. We clearly favor the first two alternatives, providing the treatment period

Table 6-10. Monthly/Maintenance Exercise Questionnaire

Name _____   Date _____

1. How satisfied are you with your progress so far in the exercise program?

       1   2   3   4   5   6   7   8   9
    Not at all satisfied   Very satisfied

2. Does this exercise program make sense to you?

       1   2   3   4   5   6   7   8   9
    Definitely NO   Definitely YES

3. Would you recommend this kind of treatment to a friend or relative who has high blood pressure?

       1   2   3   4   5   6   7   8   9
    Definitely NO   Definitely YES

4. What kind of exercise have you been doing *at home* during the past month?

    Type of Activity   *Min/Hours*   *Times Per Week*

5. Has your diet changed in any way or are you eating/drinking more/less since you began the exercise program? Yes/No? Please describe:

_____

_____

6. How confident are you that you can/will complete the *3-month exercise program* (4 times per week)?

       1   2   3   4   5   6   7   8   9
    Not at all confident   Very confident

7. How confident are you that you can/will continue exercising for 1 year

       1   2   3   4   5   6   7   8   9
    Not at all confident   Very confident

can be extended (this will take agreement from the patient, his or her physician, and the exercise program staff). We do caution those conducting any nondrug treatment for hypertension that it may not be wise, from a cardiovascular-risk-reduction perspective, to keep a hypertensive off medications for longer than 3 to 4 months. Whatever decision may be made regarding the poor responder to the exercise intervention, it should be made in close consultation with the patient's physician.

Phase II: Exercise Plateau: Early
Home Generalization

Weeks 5 to 10. Once a patient has met criteria to advance into the second phase, we assume that the exercise habit has been well enough established to allow increases in exertion to maximize the BP-lowering potential of the exercise. At this point, patients may be allowed or encouraged to exercise more predominantly in a single *mode* (e.g., treadmill/walk/jog *or* cycling) for the whole 30-minute period. This exercise should be one that is most easily generalizable to the home environment (if they have no access to a stationary bicycle, then the majority of their time should be spent on the treadmill, or in walking/jogging on a trail or course). We are also open to changes in exercise *frequency* sometimes allowing patients to gradually increase to 5 or even 6 days a week, providing they are moderate in intensity, there is at least one complete day off a week, and every other workout is a relatively easy one. We set these conditions to reduce the risk of physical and psychological aversiveness as well as the potential for injury and exercise relapse due to massing (as opposed to spacing) exercise-training sessions. Generally, 3 or 4 days is plenty, and was sufficient to produce large reductions in BP in many of our hypertensives. In some cases, we have even allowed patients to increase their exercise *duration* up to 45 minutes; however, this is allowed only for those who can easily exercise the full 30 minutes at the upper ranges of the prescribed intensity (75% to 80% maximum HR). Finally, with respect to exercise *intensity* we will, under controlled circumstances at first, allow RPE to go to 13 ("somewhat hard") or slightly above, and may let patients who have developed more fitness to go as high as 80% to 85% of their maximum HR periodically, but we studiously guard the *enjoyability* criterion of no more than two consecutive sessions in the neutral or negative range before changing the routine.

At the conclusion of the first session in Week 5, patients are informed that laboratory sessions will only be held once a week, and that we will be adding a home session to the two they are already completing. Generally, we note this at the beginning of the program, stating that if they do well and adhere properly, after the fifth week they will only need to come in once a week. Most find this reinforcing, although in some instances we have had patients request that we continue with two laboratory sessions per week.

A second reinforcer we employ, which has important implications for home generalization, consists of taking the patients out on our walking/jogging trail. They are always accompanied by an exercise leader or assistant, and sometimes even other patients. The assistant praises them frequently, and we try to choose the nicest days for the outdoor experiences.

Finally, we spend considerable time discussing and trying to enlist home social support for our patients' exercise habit and program. We encourage family members to come exercise with the hypertensive in the laboratory as well as at home. If they are unable to attend, we speak with them by phone on a regular basis to prompt, guide and reinforce their efforts at being a good "health helper."

Week 6. Similar to other weeks, we begin by reviewing the patients' *home self-monitoring records,* praising adherence as well as any improvements, while encouraging self-statements and attributions crediting their efforts in successfully mastering the exercise habit and control over their blood pressure. This is a critical stage for ensuring effective exercise adherence since the patients have just faded to only one laboratory session per week and the potential for slips and program drop-out is higher. We recommend watching very carefully for drops in enjoyment ratings, difficulties establishing a regular time and place to exercise at home, rapid increases in exercise intensity (RPE above 13 and exercise HR consistently above 80% to 85% maximum HR), or significant variability in intensity, duration and frequency. The hypertensive exercisers should be settling into somewhat of a "groove" by now, where there is some consistency in mode, time, location, frequency, and especially pacing of the exercise sessions. This session is also an excellent time to discuss fading and generalization with the patients, noting the importance to any long-term habit change of establishing and overlearning the behavior in the natural environment, while at the same time fading out the artificial, laboratory sessions. We suggest spending time problem solving with the patients, covering all the obstacles that might impinge upon the effective following of the home exercise program, and what to do when those events or situations are encountered. In any event, probably the most important feature of this beginning generalization period is to ensure continued, though less frequent, laboratory sessions, and to carefully and outwardly monitor patients' self-monitoring forms each session.

The exercise session for Week 6 will consist of at least two 15-minute periods of aerobic exercise with little or no rest, with the patient controlling workloads, treadmill, pedaling and path-walking speed, and HR monitoring. Patients may have progressed to 20 to 30 minutes without stopping and, providing this can be done easily, we encourage patients to continue beyond the 15-minute time block up to a maximum of 30 minutes. Again, we carefully monitor breathing, sweating, RPE, enjoyment and HR levels to guard against overexertion. By this time, patients should be taking their own BP at the end of each session.

Week 7. The procedures this week are similar to those for the previous week, with the addition that we invite the patient to bring family members to the final four weekly laboratory sessions (Weeks 8, 9, 10, 12). We also discuss the importance of good social support for maintaining the exercise habit, as follows:

> As we have discussed previously, good *social support* is practically essential to maintaining your exercise program at home once we fade out the laboratory sessions. What exactly do we mean by social support? Basically, we mean the active support of other people in your home and work environments in helping you both to feel good about what you are doing here *and* to actually stick with your health program. This might come in the form of pats on the back or praise when you are really doing well with your program ("Hey, way to stick with that program . . . you look so much healthier. . . . Boy, I have to admire you, I don't think I could ever do what you have done with this exercise thing!") We all know how nice that feels when someone compliments us for something we are doing or have done. It could also come in the form of encouragement when you are down or are having trouble staying on your exercise program ("you have done so well, it's okay to slip a little . . . everybody does some time or another . . . think how far you've come . . . tomorrow's a new day . . . you can do it!"). One of the very best forms of social support is to have others exercise with you. Have you noticed how much more pleasant and distracting your exercise sessions are when you talk with a fellow exerciser or with us while you are exercising? Well, that is what we are talking about. We should note that social support does not include nagging you when you slip a little or resenting your program for the time it takes away from the family or work. In fact, this negative support can often backfire and have just the opposite effect—you want to exercise even less because you feel worse because you are angry and guilty.
> We want to help you enlist positive social support so that when we are not as regularly available, others can give you the reinforcement and encouragement that you will need. First, we would like you to learn to ask others to support you by giving you "strokes" when you are doing well. Your family is an important place to start, but co-workers and friends are also excellent sources of positive strokes. Tell them what you are doing and why it is important and how they might help you with their encouragement and praise. Ask them to inquire about your program. Put a graph up on the wall of your adherence (sessions per week, or minutes of exercise per week) to your exercise program. Display it publicly so all can see and comment. Another way we have of enlisting social support is to contract with another for certain desirable things in return for achieving your exercise goals. Next week we would like you to bring your wife or a family member, or close friend, who is willing to exercise with you or, if not, at least will contract with us and

you to provide support in some form for your exercise program. How does that sound? Any questions?

Week 8. In this week, the exercise bout should be very similar to the previous week. Following resting BP measurement done by the patient, review of last session and problem solving (of self-monitoring/home exercise session adherence and performance), the goals and procedures of the exercise program are discussed with the family member or friend who was brought to the sessions by the hypertensive patient. We recommend that the patient do as much of this explaining and demonstrating to the significant other as possible. This serves to reinforce their knowledge of and personal responsibility for the exercise treatment. In addition, we suggest that the significant other exercise along with the patient. We encourage the patient, again, to show their significant other (monitored carefully by the therapist) the proper way to exercise. We pay careful attention that the helpers are not physically overextended, and we invite them back for the remainder of the sessions. We also strongly recommend that they exercise with the patient at home or work. When possible, we ask both patient and helper to sign a contract specifying the social support that will be provided, and the conditions under which it will be given (see Fig. 6–4).

Week 9. This week's session is similar to Weeks 7 and 8, and includes a formal exercise period with both the patient and family member or friend. A review of the home sessions and self-monitoring is conducted, along with problem solving for any difficulties noted by either patient or helper. Time permitting, we try to review the various exercise-adherence strategies with the patient, including reinforcement, stimulus control, cognitive distraction, enhancing enjoyability, and social support.

Week 10. The optional submaximal fitness test may then be readministered in Week 10 to assess fitness improvements, home-exercise adherence and provide feedback to the patient. The test is identical to that performed in Weeks 2 and 5, and HR results are placed on the same graph and compared (fitness improvements should be illustrated by a lower curve for lower HRs across testings). As in Week 5, the latter portion of the session includes a regular 15-to-20-minute aerobic-exercise bout.

The same criteria shown in Week 5 should be met before patients are recommended for the final program fading and generalization to a home exercise format. One additional criterion is that their resting BP should be in the normotensive range by this time ($< 140/90$ mm Hg). If BP is still in the hypertensive range, and has not shown signs of lowering, then referral back to their physician for medication should be strongly considered. It may be that 10 weeks of aerobic training is insufficient to lower BP in that individual, and patient and physician may vote for extended exercise training. We found that in over 90% of our patients, 8 to 10 weeks was sufficient. If the adherence and fitness-improvement criteria are not met, but BP is in or near the normotensive range (and has dropped at least 5 mm Hg DBP), then continuation in the weekly laboratory session phase should be extended if at all possible until these criteria (especially the 80% adherence floor) are met.

Phase III: Final Home-Generalization Training

This last, relatively brief treatment phase assumes that BP has been effectively controlled *and* that good laboratory and home adherence to the program has been demonstrated. Patients are faded to once every 2 weeks for 2 sessions (exercising 4 times on their own during off weeks), followed by optional monthly laboratory sessions for 3 months and 3-month follow-ups for a year. We recommend phoning patients or their significant other/helper at the midpoint between these less frequent laboratory sessions (i.e., on off weeks) to detect and intervene on any problems early, to reinforce maintenance, and to lend general support and encouragement.

Week 12. Initially, self-monitoring and home-exercise performance is carefully reviewed for the previous 2 weeks, and any problems are discussed and remedied. A normal exercise session of 30 minutes is then conducted following resting BP measurement, in a fashion similar to previous sessions. Four home-exercise sessions per week are then prescribed for the coming 2 weeks, and any questions answered. During exercising, the final teaching component is presented and discussed. This is *relapse innoculation*. An example of how this might be presented is as follows:

> The final skill that should help you maintain your exercise program concerns how to deal with those almost-inevitable slips in regular exercising on your own. Remember, at the beginning of this program we discussed the importance of just showing up, and not making excuses for not coming for your exercise session. We also discussed the many life events that seem to be related to failures to exercise—such as sickness, moving, injuries, loss of exercise partners, stress, or loss in motivation. One of the prime events connected with stopping exercising is "graduating" from a formal exercise program such as this one. That is why we have concentrated so much on establishing your exercise program at home, too.

The best way to maximize your chances of sticking to your exercise program is to rehearse what to do when you have one of these lapses in your home-exercise program. This will enable you to get back on your program without having to start all over again in a formal clinic program. We know that most people who begin an exercise program will stop at some point, even if briefly for illness or injury. The problem is a good number of those will never successfully get back on their program. Thus, the question for most is not *whether* they fall off their exercise program, but rather *how to respond* when they do. Research in the field of health-behavior change suggests that the following may be helpful:

1. Admit that the slip has occurred, and take responsibility for it, without blaming or feeling guilty. It happened, it's quite normal—now what is the best way to cope with it? It's a good idea to call a friend, your exercise helper, or us, and discuss objectively what can be done.

2. Set an immediate plan to exercise within a day or two. Write your plan down and discuss it with another. Ask them to follow up and ask you whether you actually followed through with your plan. Your plan should include: what, when, where, for how long, and with whom to exercise. If you want, call us. We can assist you with finding a partner, or offering our laboratory and a special assistant to help you.

3. Arrange to meet another for this "comeback" session. This should be someone who wants you to exercise and would like to help you. Ideally, it should be one who would exercise with you. If you get stuck, call us. We'll help.

4. No matter what, show up at the appointed time and place . . . no matter how you feel. You are likely to feel bad, and to want to do anything but exercise. Resist this self-defeating impulse, and gently but firmly force yourself to go out and exercise at least once for even a very short period.

5. On the day before the planned exercise, lay out your exercise things where you will stumble over them, and carry them with you during the day (so no matter where you are, you can go prepared at the appointed time). Wear your exercise clothes as early in the comeback day as possible. Another good idea is to have your partner call you and/or pick you up to further prompt you.

6. When you exercise, make sure it is easy and enjoyable. If you have not exercised in over 10 days or so, exercise at about 50% (intensity, duration) or less of your last exercise session. Make certain it is easy and enjoyable. Your HR for your first few sessions back should not exceed 75% of the maximum, and your RPE should be less than 12 as a general guideline. You might also pick a convenient place that has distractions and a pleasant environment and don't think about the exercise when you do exercise.

7. Reinforce your showing up to exercise. A good idea is to plan a special reward, such as a back rub from your wife or a special dinner or movie, following your exercise session. No matter how little you actually do, reward yourself—you are back on the road to exercise-habit recovery and you deserve praise and rewards! For best results, try to do this for several sessions.

8. If you have stopped self-monitoring and tracking (e.g., graphing and posting) exercise data, then go back to this.

Okay let's discuss this now, relating it to your situation, and what is likely to happen to you and how we might best plan for your return to exercising. Let's go through some examples that you think of . . . Great . . . any questions?

Week 14. This last formal treatment session should consist of a 30-minute exercise bout, following resting HR and BP measurement and self-monitoring review and problem solving. A review of learning components should be held during the exercise session, including (especially) relapse innoculation. A long-term contract should be signed in which the patient agrees to attend follow-up sessions, and to continue to fill out self-monitoring forms. We recommend that this be done in conjunction with the family member/helper. At this point, discuss with the patients their exercise maintenance and follow-up.

Phase IV: Maintenance and Follow-up

We recommend *monthly maintenance sessions* for approximately the next 3 months, with telephone contact made at each 2-week mark to assess progress and problems. This could then be followed by *3-month follow-up* visits for the next year (again, with phone contact made at the midpoint between visits). We also suggest, to those professionals and programs who can arrange for this, or who might perform it themselves, that submaximal-exercise testing, such as the one we use, be conducted at the maintenance/follow-up sessions, at least every 3 to 6 months.

Obviously, resting BP should always be obtained at these visits, but a good supplement or minimal alternative is to have patients return to you their signed BP records from their physicians, nurse, or public health clinic. We also recommend home BP assessments be conducted on about a weekly basis by the patients. Those measures should be recorded in the self-monitoring forms, and then carefully examined at all maintenance and follow-up visits. Regular physician visits should also continue, according to the schedule requested by their physician, and formal contact should be maintained between psychologist or other nonmedical therapy providers. We recommend a personal letter and written progress reports be sent to their physician or health clinic; if this is not acknowledged in some way, then it is appropriate and desirable to call or directly contact the patient's physician.

For patients whose BP rises into the hypertensive range, more frequent clinic visits are recommended (every other week) until BP is reduced once again, or until three consecutive high-blood-pressure readings are registered. In the latter case, referral can be made for drug therapy, or exercise and other behavioral interventions can be stepped up. In any event, patients should be monitored and followed very carefully because some may feel "cured" and discontinue both their exercise regimen and their medical follow-up.

SOME FINAL CONSIDERATIONS

What about different kinds of exercise? In our laboratory we caution hypertensives against anaerobic or isometric exercises that involve explosive movements or isolation of one particular muscle group without rhythmic movement. These activities are not likely to benefit the cardiovascular system (ACSM, 1980) and may be associated with rapid spiking of blood pressure. For these reasons we are generally opposed to this form of exercise for hypertensives and would recommend against it.

Occasionally, we have individuals ask us if circuit training, or lifting lighter weights more rapidly, and quickly "circuiting" to the next machine (e.g., Nautilus equipment), is an aerobic, cardiovascular workout, that might help their blood pressure. Unfortunately, to date no good studies have supported this contention. We instruct our patients that although circuit training is not as potentially harmful as heavy weight lifting, and that it can indeed increase strength and flexibility, it will not likely help lower their blood pressure.

Another question that is often asked is: "Does routine, low-level physical activity such as walking to work, taking the stairs, and so forth, help? The answer is yes and no. These activities are generally not done for long enough periods to provide aerobic benefit or blood-pressure lowering, per se. They can, however, help to reinforce the patients' active lifestyle that we are promoting, and may serve as excellent prompts for greater levels of exercise. Further, for the most unfit (e.g., very obese smoker who has never exercised), increasing routine physical activities can be an excellent place to begin in shaping them gradually toward the minimum aerobic-training level that is necessary for cardiovascular benefit, and especially for blood-pressure control. In these cases especially we would recommend issuing pedometers to track daily walking mileage (digital, to tenths of miles, are best). Particularly in individuals who are not able to exercise very much at first, the pedometer will show them their increases in tenths of miles, which often is highly reinforcing feedback (so reinforcing, we might add, that when our first shipment of pedometers turned up missing, we tracked them to our supply department where a number of the employees had been "testing them," drastically increasing *their* activity levels for several weeks!).

Finally, we insist that the programmed aerobic exercises we conduct ultimately be the patients' primary physical activity. In other words, we train patients that it is all right to play doubles tennis or golf, or lift light weights, but these should be done only *after* their prescribed aerobic regimen is completed for that day (e.g., a brisk walk 30 minutes before the golf game). For the Type A/highly competitive individual we attempt to discourage the use of competitive activities to fulfill the exercise prescription (though, as noted, they might come on top of the regular program of exercise), because we are attempting to modify the type, quantity, and quality of exercise so that a lifetime habit of enjoyable and effective activity is incorporated into their lifestyles—not geared to any competitive goal. We believe this approach is important in facilitating adherence to their baseline, most beneficial activity, the aerobic exercise.

Exercise Equipment and Setting Considerations

It is not essential that the health professional or psychologist have an exercise laboratory, but it is desirable. We recommend one or more stationary bicycle ergometers (a fancier exercycle with workload settings). These can be purchased for around $200 to $600 (we suggest brands such as Monarch, Schwinn, Bodyguard and Tunturi). A motorized treadmill, although it is a very nice addition, is much more expensive (around $5000 to $15,000). We would encourage psychologists and others to use, as consultants, exercise physiologists and physicians (many cardiologists, internists and others now are involved in the prescription of exercise and fitness programs for their patients). Finally, there are many exercise facilities that might welcome collaboration with psychologists and others who want to treat their patients through exercise.

Exercise-Program Training for the Non Expert

We recommend that health professionals considering employing exercise as a mode of therapy with their hypertensives seek specialized training in exercise testing, prescription, and training. This recommendation is made to (a) ensure the safety of the patients, (b) protect the psychologist or other professional from liability should some problem arise, and (c) maximize the probabilities that the very best exercise program will be developed and provided to the hypertensive patient. Excellent training and certification is conducted through the

American College of Sports Medicine (ACSM), P.O. Box 1440, Indianapolis, IN 46206; telephone (317) 637-9200. The ACSM, and other organizations such as the Cooper Clinic and Institute for Aerobics Research in Dallas, provide 1-to-2-week training courses throughout the year in exercise testing, prescription, and program implementation. We strongly encourage interested persons to contact them for further information and course schedules. We do not suggest that exercise therapy be conducted with hypertensives without both regular consultation with medical and/or exercise physiology specialists and ACSM or similar training.

A Final Note of Caution

As in other nonpharmacological methods of controlling this serious disease, caution should be used so that hypertensives are not permitted to independently drop out of treatment without systematic follow-up and/or medical referral. As we suggested earlier, without adequate instructions and follow-up, individuals may be likely to believe they are "cured" once BP has been temporarily controlled (a feeling some of our patients have expressed) and discontinue not only the exercise and other behavioral regimens but also their medication-taking and physician contact.

Indeed, while working in our clinic we saw a number of previously untreated individuals who have through a regular program of exercise achieved controlled diastolic blood pressures; still others have been able to reduce or discontinue their medication. Yet, is clear that exercise treatment can only help control blood pressure as long as the exercise prescription is properly followed. Our preliminary follow-up data and the two-subject studies suggest that a return to hypertensive blood pressures will generally occur within several weeks of discontinuing or drastically reducing (i.e., once per week average or less) the aerobic regimen. It is possible, however, that the longer an individual with high blood pressure maintains blood-pressure control through exercising, the longer it will take for blood pressures to return to hypertensive levels. This same effect may also appear in patients who have had their blood pressures controlled for an extended period of time by pharmaco-therapy, in whom medications are faded out, and this period may be an ideal one for instituting a behavioral regimen of exercise—and perhaps diet and stress management—to maintain lowered blood pressure. Our final chapter will address this issue, along with other aspects of integrating nondrug approaches to treating hypertension.

Chapter 7

Dietary Interventions with Hypertension

Diet interventions are the oldest type of behavioral intervention for hypertension, dating back at least to the 1920s. Today, both weight-reduction and low-sodium diets are widely accepted, either as primary treatment or in combination with pharmacotherapy (Subcommittee on Nonpharmacological Therapy, 1986). Although diet therapy has been shown to be very effective and capable of significantly reducing the medication requirements for many hypertensives, compliance is often poor (Glanz, 1980). For this reason, patients will often be referred for behavioral interventions, which can help them adhere to dietary-treatment programs.

The dietary-treatment-team. Diet therapy, like exercise, is an area in which most psychologists have little or no formal training. It is therefore important to recognize and make use of the expertise of registered dietitians and other specialists who have the knowledge and experience to carefully assess patients' nutritional status and instruct them on appropriate dietary changes. Without this kind of guidance, patients may adopt new maladaptive diet habits, such as inadequate intake of iron or calcium, as they attempt to meet the goals of weight and/or sodium reduction (Nowalk & Wing, 1985). In medical center settings, patients are usually referred to a clinical dietitian on staff for diet instruction and nutrition teaching. In outpatient settings, physicians or medical groups may employ a dietitian to perform this service. If your patient needs diet instructions and the referring physician does not have a consulting dietitian, the nearest university medical center, the state dietetic association, or the local affiliate of the American Heart Association can suggest someone who is qualified to work with hypertensive patients. We suggest working closely with the dietitians who provide the dietary instructions. In fact, co-therapy in a group format with psychologist and dietitian co-leaders can be a particularly effective approach and has been used in a number of clinical and research programs.

While moderate sodium restriction and sensible weight reduction are unlikely to have adverse effects on patients, it is also important to consult with the patient's physician before working on any diet changes. It is helpful to know the physician's beliefs about the importance of diet changes, verify whether a specific diet has been prescribed, determine whether the patient has already been referred for diet instruction, and find out if there are any medical restrictions, such as limitations on physical exercise or use of salt substitutes, which would affect the range of behavioral interventions available for the patient. It may also be necessary to discuss the physician's role in assessing progress toward the dietary goals, such as ordering urine sodium analyses.

Family members and other individuals who wish to improve their diets along with the patient but who do not need a weight-reduction or sodium-restricted diet can be advised to follow the American Heart Association Diet, "An Eating Plan for Healthy Americans." This is a "heart-healthy" diet plan that provides for all the necessary nutrients while reducing excess calories, sodium, and total fat and cholesterol. The American Heart Association diet is described in one of many excellent brochures published by this association for the benefit of heart patients and the public. The American Heart Association also publishes several very good cookbooks and some affiliates hold cooking classes which can be helpful to your hypertensive patients. We suggest a call or visit to the local office to find out what is available.

EVIDENCE FOR THE EFFECTIVENESS OF DIET IN THE TREATMENT OF HYPERTENSION

The two major dietary treatments of hypertension are weight-reduction and low-sodium diets. Obesity and high salt intake are related to high blood pressure in studies of disease risk in populations and there is growing evidence from experimental studies that reducing calorie and sodium intake can significantly lower blood pressure in many patients.

Weight-Reduction Diets

Weight and blood pressure. Numerous epidemiological studies have documented the correlation between obesity and blood pressure for children, adolescents, and adults in Western cultures. Adult hypertensives average about 30% over ideal weight and other obesity-related metabolic disorders such as non-insulin-dependent diabetes and hyperlipidemia are also common in these patients. Although not all obese individuals develop hypertension, the association is a close one at all age ranges and it is thought that the two conditions may be genetically linked (Sims, 1982). The physiological mechanisms that produce hypertension in overweight individuals are complex, and may include increased sodium retention related to hyperinsulinemia, maladaptive catecholamine responses related to excess caloric intake, and derangements of steroid metabolism (Sims, 1982). Although the mechanisms are not yet fully understood, many studies have already shown that weight loss is associated with a fall in blood pressure in a large proportion of hypertensive persons (Subcommittee on Nonpharmacological Therapy, 1986). Hovell (1982) reviewed 21 experimental studies and concluded that an average weight loss of 11.7 kg (25.74 lb) produced reductions in blood pressure of 21/13 mm Hg. In other words, diastolic blood pressure was reduced about 1 mm Hg for each kg (2.2 lb) of weight loss. It is now generally agreed that weight reduction should be the first step of therapy for many obese hypertensive patients (Berchtold, Jorgens, Kemmer, & Berger, 1982; Sims, 1982).

Weight versus sodium reduction. A decrease in caloric intake is usually accompanied by a decrease in salt intake, so which is responsible for the effect on blood pressure? Several studies have now produced good evidence that the blood-pressure reductions obtained with weight loss are independent of the level of sodium intake. Reisin and his colleagues in Israel (Reisin et al., 1978) put 81 obese hypertensive patients on low-calorie diets (1200 calories for males, 1000 calories for females up to 20% overweight; 1000 calories and 800 calories, respectively for males and females over 20% overweight). Patients were encouraged to eat freely various pickled vegetables and other low-calorie salty foods and drink at least 2500 ml (2½ quarts) of fluids daily. After 2 months, patients had lost more than 20 pounds. The weight loss was accompanied by an average drop in systolic blood pressure of 26 mm Hg and a drop in diastolic blood pressure of 20 mm Hg. Reisin et al. pointed out that, although blood pressure changes were correlated with weight loss, the individual response of blood pressure to weight change was highly variable, even among patients with similar baseline blood pressures. However, all except 2 of the 81 patients showed a reduction of at least 8 mm Hg in either systolic or diastolic blood pressures, and 74 showed reductions of this magnitude in both measures.

In a second study controlling for sodium intake, Eliahou, Ianina, Gaon, Schochat, & Modan (1981) put 212 hypertensive patients who were at least 10% overweight on a balanced low-calorie (about 1100 calories per day) diet. All patients were encouraged to eat as much salt as they wished, and their urine sodium analyses showed that average sodium intake did not change during the diet. Although 42% of the patients failed to comply with the program requirements, of those who did, about 80% were able to achieve normal blood pressure even though most were still more than 10% overweight. Through regression analyses, Eliahou's research group predicted that two-thirds of the patients could achieve normal blood pressures by losing only one half of their excess weight.

Behavioral diet-change programs. The success of behavioral treatment for obesity has not gone unnoticed by hypertension researchers, and behavioral psychologists have contributed to the development of dietary-change programs used in recent clinical trials. A study conducted by Wing at the University of Pittsburgh School of Medicine (Wing, Caggiula, Nowalk, Koeske, Lee, & Langford (1984) assessed the independence of weight and dietary electrolyte interventions as part of a feasibility study for the Dietary Intervention Study in Hypertension (DISH). In the preliminary study, 52 mild hypertensives were randomly assigned to either a weight-reduction or sodium/potassium-change diet protocol. Both interventions were conducted in group formats with behavior therapist and nutritionist co-leaders. At the end of the 8-week program, weight-reduction patients had lost an average of 9.61 pounds but showed no significant change in sodium and potassium excretion. (Electrolyte changes for patients in the sodium-intervention group will be discussed in the next section.) These weight changes, although modest, were associated with significant blood pressure reductions, averaging 13.9/7.7 mm Hg.

Jeffery and his colleagues at the University of Minnesota have also been actively involved in the development of behavioral dietary change programs for the prevention and treatment of hypertension. In one study conducted over two years with 93 overweight adult men who had labile blood-pressure elevations, these researchers compared group and individual counseling formats for a weight-and-sodium-reduction program (Jeffery, Gillum, Gerber, Jacobs, Elmer, & Prineas, 1983). The weight and sodium reduction components were introduced sequentially over 20 weeks. Participants lost an average of about 6 pounds and, as expected, the results showed no differences between individual and group treatment formats. Significant changes in systolic and diastolic blood pressure were associated with the weight and sodium changes: 9.1/4.8 mm Hg for group treatment and 7.0/5.4 mm Hg for individual treatment patients.

Use of appetite suppressants. Although sufficient to lower blood pressure, the average weight losses of 10 to 20 pounds in behavioral programs are inadequate for persons who need to lose 50 pounds or more for other reasons. Pharmacotherapy with appetite-suppressing drugs can speed up the rate of weight loss and achieved some popularity in the 1970s. Stunkard et al. (1980) conducted an important study comparing behavior therapy, pharmacotherapy, and a combination of these two treatments with a patient population including 57 hypertensives. After 6 months of treatment, patients who received only behavior therapy lost 10.9 kg (23.9 lb), those who received the appetite suppressant fenfluramine alone lost 14.5 kg (31.9 lb), and those who received the combined treatment lost 15.3 kg (33.7 lb). Type of treatment had no independent effect on blood pressure, but unmedicated mild hypertensives showed the greatest improvement (a drop of 14.5 mm Hg diastolic). Medicated patients showed a decrease of 5.7 mm Hg associated with the weight loss and one third of them were able to reduce or stop their medications. The blood pressure changes were maintained moderately well in the year following treatment, even though patients regained about half the weight they had lost. The most significant finding for this study, however, was that weight regain was highly dependent on type of treatment. The one year follow-up showed a "striking reversal" of the initial effects of treatment: The behavior therapy patients regained only 1.9 kg, which was markedly less than the pharmacotherapy patients (8.2 kg) and the combined therapy patients (10.7 kg). Because previous research findings had also indicated that weight losses induced by pharmacotherapy are not maintained at 1 year (Ost & Gotestam, 1976), appetite suppressants cannot be recommended for dietary treatment of hypertensives.

Rapid weight loss with very-low-calorie diets. In the search for methods to improve total weight losses, very-low-calorie diets are now being used with increasing frequency to treat moderate and severe obesity (patients 60% or more overweight). These diets, which supply only about 300 to 400 calories per day, have the advantage of producing rapid weight losses of 20 kg or more. The rapid weight loss and lack of hunger helps maintain the motivation of the patient. In contrast to the "liquid protein" diets, which were associated with a number of deaths, the very-low-calorie diets appear to be safe when limited to 3 months or less and when used with careful medical supervision (Wadden, Stunkard, & Brownell, 1983). Significant blood-pressure decreases accompany the weight loss for most patients (Tuck, Sowers, Dornfeld, Kledzick, & Maxwell, 1981). Unfortunately, clinical observations indicate that the weight lost on very-low-calorie diets is typically regained fairly rapidly and one of the most important questions for current research is whether behavior therapy can help prevent the weight regain (Wadden et al., 1983). Recall that Stunkard et al. (1980) found that patients receiving a combination of pharmacotherapy and behavior therapy actually had a poorer outcome after 1 year than those who received behavior therapy alone.

Wadden and Stunkard (1986) have recently reported the results of a controlled study assessing the effectiveness of very-low-calorie diet, behavior therapy, and a combination of the two treatments for patients 70% to 93% overweight. At the end of treatment, subjects in the diet-alone group had lost 31 pounds, those in behavior therapy alone had lost 31.5 pounds, and those in the combined treatment had lost 42.5 pounds. There were no significant differences among the groups for blood pressure reductions, which averaged 11 mm Hg systolic and 8.7 mm Hg diastolic. At the 1-year follow-up, the diastolic blood pressures remained significantly lower than at baseline, but the systolic pressures did not. By this time, many subjects in all conditions had regained part of the weight they had lost. On average, the patients who received the very-low-calorie diet alone regained two thirds of the weight they had lost, and not a single one remained within 5 pounds of end-of-treatment weight. However, 44% of the behavior-therapy-alone and 29% of the combined-treatment subjects regained less than 5 pounds during the year. The results of this study provide some of the most impressive evidence yet of the effectiveness of behavior-therapy-alone in the treatment of obesity, and support previous observations that the very-low-calorie diets, at least when used alone, do not produce lasting weight losses.

Long-term effects of dietary intervention: The Chicago Coronary Prevention Evaluation Program. One of the most impressive demonstrations of the long-term effectiveness of nutritional and other lifestyle interventions for hypertension was the Chicago Coronary Prevention Evaluation Program (Stamler, Farinaro, Mojonnier, Hall, Moss, & Stamler, 1980). The CPEP had the objective of controlling multiple coronary disease risk factors (obesity, hypertension, hypercholesterolemia, cigarette smoking, and physical inactivity) in high-risk men aged 40 to 59 years at entry. Sixty-seven of the 333 subjects who completed the 5-year program were unmedicated hypertensives who were 15% or more overweight at baseline. These men were advised to reduce their calorie intake to about 1750 calories per day and to engage in light exercise at least 3 times each week. After 5 years, they maintained average weight losses of 11.7 pounds and showed significant reductions in blood pressure, heart rate, and serum cholesterol levels. It is important to note that moderate losses (5% to 6% of body weight over the 5-year period) were sufficient to produce the therapeutic effect.

Dietary prevention of relapse after drug treatment of hypertension. In the only study of its kind, the Dietary Intervention Study in Hypertension (DISH) (Langford et al., 1985) evaluated whether weight-loss and low-sodium diet interventions could reduce the relapse rate for hypertensive patients taken off medications. This important clinical trial included almost 500 patients who were followed for approximately 1 year after drug therapy was discontinued. All patients had well-controlled blood pressure during a previous drug study (the Hypertension Detection and Follow-Up (HDFP) study). Obese patients were randomized into weight reduction, sodium restriction, or control (no diet) groups, while normal-weight patients were randomized into sodium-restriction or control groups. After 32 weeks, the overweight patients showed an average reduction of 5% of their body weight (about 10 lb) and maintained this reduction to the end of the study. Weight reduction significantly improved the likelihood of patients' blood pressures remaining under control without medications. At the end of the study, 60% of all the weight-reduction diet patients were controlled without drugs, as compared with only 35% of the overweight patients who had received no dietary intervention. Success rates for patients with only mild blood pressure elevations were even better—72% of the overweight mild hypertensives on weight loss diets had normal blood pressure without medications after 1 year. The results for the sodium-restriction intervention were also impressive and will be discussed in the next section.

Low-Salt or Sodium-Restricted Diets

Salt and sodium. A large proportion of the sodium in Western diets comes from added salt; therefore sodium-restricted diets are essentially low-salt diets. Because different clinicians and researchers use different terminology for measuring sodium, it is necessary to be familiar with the common terms. Ordinary table salt is sodium chloride, which is about 40% sodium by weight. A gram is a unit of weight; there are about 28 grams in 1 ounce and 5.5 grams in a teaspoon. A milliEquivalent (mEq) is a unit of chemical activity and is useful for understanding the sodium ion's activity in the body. One gram of sodium chloride (salt) contains about 17 mEq of sodium; one teaspoon of salt contains a little less than 100 mEq of sodium. Besides table salt, baking soda (sodium bicarbonate), MSG (monosodium glutamate), and preservatives in processed foods are the main sources of sodium in most diets.

Sodium and blood pressure. In cross-cultural studies, it has been shown that populations with low sodium or salt intake generally do not have a high incidence of hypertension, whereas populations with extremely high sodium intake have a higher incidence of hypertension. These findings are often cited to support the hypothesis that the sodium-intake characteristic of modern Western cultures (about 100 to 250 mEq/day, which is about 10 times more than the biological requirement) is an important cause of hypertension. The findings of cross-cultural studies must be interpreted cautiously, however, because the populations differ on many important variables other than sodium intake (Page, 1983).

Clinical trials. Athough there had been earlier reports of blood pressure reductions through sodium restriction, real interest in this kind of intervention was not aroused until the 1940s when Kempner reported substantial decreases in blood pressure with the "rice and fruit diet" (Kopelman & Dzau, 1985; Langford, 1982). However, this diet was too difficult for most people to follow. More recent controlled studies have demonstrated that moderate and acceptable levels of sodium restriction can lower blood pressure.

One important, well-controlled study was conducted by MacGregor and his colleagues in London (MacGregor et al., 1982). In this study, 19 hypertensive patients were followed for 2 months without medication and then given instructions by the study dietitian for a 60 to 80 mEq sodium diet. For most patients, the salt intake was reduced primarily by not adding salt at the table or in cooking, and by avoiding high-sodium foods. Patients who did not think they could comply with the diet were excluded. After 2 weeks on the sodium-restricted diet, the patients were entered into a double-blind crossover study. During this part of the the study they received, in random order, for 4 weeks each, either supplemental sodium to bring their total intake to baseline levels or a placebo. When the data were analyzed, the results showed that although there was considerable variation in individual patients' responses, the mean blood pressures were 7.1 mm Hg lower during the placebo (low-sodium) phase of the study. Like most of the sodium-restriction evaluations published thus far, the number of subjects was small and the intervention was for a very short period of time.

In a longer term study, Morgan and his colleagues (Morgan, Adam, Gillies, Wilson, Morgan, & Carney, 1978) treated 31 mildly hypertensive patients for 2 years with a moderately salt-restricted diet. The diet instructions were designed to bring patients' total sodium intake down to about 70 to 100 mEq per day. On the average, patients instructed in the low-salt diet reduced their diastolic blood pressure by 7.3 mm Hg, which was comparable to the results for other similar patients treated with diuretic drugs. The authors noted that the blood-pressure improvements were achieved in spite of less than optimal compliance: Although the prescribed diet was at a 100 mEq sodium level, patients actually reduced their sodium intake from about 200 mEq to about 160 mEq.

In a study described earlier, Wing et al. (1984) carefully examined goal achievement by weight-reduction and sodium/potassium-intervention patients. After 8 weeks of treatment, sodium/potassium patients decreased their average sodium excretion from 169 mEq per day to 108 mEq per day and increased their potassium excretion from 76 mEq to 82 mEq per day. Only a small percent, however, were able to meet the target levels of less than 70 mEq sodium and more than 100 mEq potassium daily. (In contrast, over half the weight-reduction patients were able to meet their goals.) Despite this difficulty in meeting the target levels, blood pressures dropped significantly, by 6.2/4.1 mm Hg, for the electrolyte-change participants. In discussing their results, Wing et al. (1984) noted that, at this point, we do not know if it is the absolute level of sodium or potassium, the ratio of these in the diet, or the percentage of change that is important in controlling blood pressure.

Dietary prevention of relapse with sodium restriction. The results of DISH demonstrated that a sodium-restricted diet can reduce the probability of relapse after antihypertensive medications are discontinued in both overweight and normal-weight patients. Overweight participants instructed in a low-salt diet reduced their sodium intake from 158 mEq to 106 mEq, and nonoverweight participants reduced theirs from 130 mEq to 96 mEq. As in previous studies (Morgan et al., 1978; Wing et al., 1984), both groups fell short of reaching the goal of < 70 mEq sodium per day. Nevertheless, the sodium reductions significantly improved the patients' chances of having blood pressure controlled without medication. At the end of the year, normal-weight hypertensives who had reduced their sodium intake had a 53% success rate (which was similar to the rate for overweight patients who had lost weight). Those with only mild blood pressure elevations showed the best results of all—with sodium restriction, 78% were still controlled without medications at the 1-year evaluation (which was 20% better than their control group).

Potassium, Calcium, and other
Dietary Interventions

Because it is almost impossible to devise a very-low-sodium diet that is not also high in potassium, another explanation for the very low blood pressures found in cultural groups with low sodium intake is their high potassium intake. There have now been a few controlled trials of potassium supplementation in hypertensive humans; however, the results have not been very promising: changes in blood pressure, if any, have been small and variable (Subcommittee on Nonpharmacologic Therapy, 1986). In a recent, randomized, short-term study, Richards et al. (1984) evaluated the blood pressure responses of 12 patients to three diet regimens: (a) a control diet (180 mEq sodium), (b) a sodium-restricted diet (80 mEq sodium), and (c) a potassium-supplemented diet (200 mEq potassium per day). The patients stayed on each diet for 4 weeks and the order of the 3 diets was randomized. As in the MacGregor et al. (1982) study, not all patients had lower blood pressures on the sodium-restricted diet. In Richards' study, 7 of the 12 patients had lower blood pressures, but 5 had higher blood pressures on the low-salt diet, and the average change was only 4/3 mm Hg lower (not significant). Potassium supplementation produced variable changes in blood pressure, and the overall mean difference of $-1/.8$ mm Hg was also not significant.

McCarron and others (McCarron, Morris, Henry, & Stanton, 1984) have recently called attention to data suggesting a relationship between calcium intake and blood pressure. The interpretation of these data has generated a good deal of controversy, and researchers are now studying the effects of calcium supplements on blood pressure. Others are looking at the role of magnesium and trace elements and at the effects of variations in dietary fat, fiber, protein, and carbohydrates. At this point, it is too early to say whether changes in any of these dietary constituents has a therapeutic effect on blood pressure. Most researchers believe that, at best, only subgroups of hypertensives will benefit from changes in these dietary components (Subcommittee on Nonpharmacological Therapy, 1986). Since potassium- and calcium-supplemented diets and other dietary changes must still be considered experimental, they will not be discussed further in this chapter.

Summary of Results of Controlled Studies
of Weight and Sodium Reduction

Weight loss is a very effective method of reducing blood pressure. In general, the research shows that weight losses of as little as 10 to 20 pounds produce significant decreases in blood pressure for many patients, although some patients may reduce more than 20 pounds without a blood-pressure reduction (Berchtold et al., 1982). Even if blood pressure fails to improve, weight reduction can bring about favorable changes in other cardiovascular-disease risk factors. Weight reduction is therefore recommended for all obese hypertensives (Berchtold et al., 1982; Subcommittee on Nonpharmacological Therapy, 1986). Behavior therapy has a good track record for weight and blood-pressure reduction in hypertensive patients. Although appetite suppressants and very-low-calorie diets produce more rapid weight loss, the available data indicate that, for lasting weight loss, appetite suppressants should be avoided and that very-low-calorie diets should be used only in combination with behavior therapy (Stunkard et al., 1980; Wadden & Stunkard, 1986).

In contrast to weight reduction, there have been relatively few well-controlled studies on the effects of moderate sodium restriction in hypertensive patients. At this time, it appears that moderate levels of sodium restriction can result in clinically significant blood-pressure reduction, but not for all patients. The current thinking is that most likely only a subset of hypertensives, perhaps 30 to 50%, benefit from sodium restriction (Laragh & Pecker, 1983). It is not possible to predict in advance who will benefit from sodium restriction, but because lowering salt intake has little potential for harm, it is generally agreed that a trial of sodium restriction is an appropriate intervention for most hypertensive patients (Subcommittee on Nonpharmacological Therapy, 1986). Behavioral techniques have been used successfully to help patients lower sodium intake in small-group studies (e.g., Jeffery et al., 1983; Wing et al., 1984) and in large clinical trials (Langford et al., 1985).

Additional research is needed to help clarify nutritional influences on the development and treatment of hypertension, in particular for mild and borderline hypertensives (Horan et al., 1985). Clinical trials now in progress will soon provide some of the needed data. The Hypertension Prevention Trial (HPT) is evaluating the feasibility of inducing sustained changes (for at least 2 years) in sodium, potassium, and caloric intake of nonhypertensive men and women (Hypertension Prevention Trial Research Group, in press) and the Trial of Antihypertensive Interventions and Management (TAIM) will provide information about the relative efficacy of drug and dietary therapy for hypertensives.

Results of Dietary Treatment by the Present Authors

Two of us (PMD and JEM) have been involved in the clinical dietary treatment of hypertensive patients for more than 7 years. Because most of the patients referred to us are "problem" clinic patients whose various medications, including antihypertensive therapy, are being adjusted every few weeks, it is often not possible for us to evaluate the role of dietary intervention alone in improved treatment outcome. On occasion, however, patients referred to us have had no changes in medication for 2 months or more, and with these cases we can observe that the results of our dietary interventions are very consistent with those of published controlled studies.

Weight reduction seems to be the most powerful dietary treatment for hypertension and most of our diet patients are referred for behavioral therapy of obesity. We evaluated the results of our weight-reduction program for one series of 9 mild hypertensive patients treated for 4 months with no changes in medication. (These patients were given no specific instructions concerning salt intake.) Four of the patients were medicated and had diastolic blood pressures below 90 mm Hg when they started the weight-reduction program. Five were unmedicated and their diastolic blood pressures ranged from 90 to 105 mm Hg. All changes in exercise for these patients were within the context of the weight-loss effort. Table 7–1 shows the weight, systolic, and diastolic blood pressure changes for these patients from baseline to the end of treatment. These results are similar to those in the controlled studies, showing an approximate reduction of 1 pound per week of treatment and a reduction in diastolic blood pressure of about 1 mm Hg for each kilogram of weight lost. Sodium intake is not routinely evaluated for our weight-reduction patients, so we were not able to determine the effect of the dietary change on sodium intake.

For our patients, sodium restriction has always been part of a more comprehensive diet (and often exercise) program. Table 7–2 presents the results for 11 hypertensive and/or cardiac patients who were followed for 3 months without medication changes. All were prescribed a combination weight-reduction, 87 mEq sodium-restricted diet, although the prescribed caloric restriction varied from 1200 calories/day to 1800 calories/day. You may note that the initial average sodium level for our patients is high compared to those reported in the controlled studies; this reflects the liberal use of sodium in the local diet. As a

Table 7-1. Authors' Results from Weight Reduction Diets for Mild Hypertensives

	Baseline	Posttreatment	Change
Weight, lb	213.3	196.9	16.4
Systolic BP, mm Hg	149	127	22
Diastolic BP, mm Hg	92	84	8

Table 7-2. Authors' Results for Sodium Restriction with Weight
Reduction

	Baseline	Posttreatment	Change
Sodium, mEq/24 hr	203.2	132.3	70.9
Weight, lb	202.4	192.6	10.3
Systolic BP, mm Hg	136.3	126.1	12.5
Diastolic BP, mm Hg	97.6	85.1	12.5

result, even after substantial reduction, the average sodium intake for these patients remained well above the goal level. The average blood-pressure reductions (2.7 mm Hg per kg of weight loss) were greater than those we observed with weight reduction alone.

REDUCING WEIGHT AND SODIUM: A 10-WEEK PLAN FOR INITIATING DIETARY CHANGE

This plan for dietary intervention contains the basic treatment components that can help patients begin losing weight and achieve a moderately restricted (87 mEq or 2 gram) daily sodium intake. The plan requires modification if the prescribed level of sodium restriction is greater than 87 mEq per day, if the patient wishes to use the food-exchange system rather than count calories, or if the patient cannot increase physical activity.

Evaluating Adherence to the Program

Adherence and outcome. Sometimes patients and clinicians mistakenly assume that changes in blood pressure after diet instruction are directly related to dietary adherence. As a result, the physician (or other health professional) may criticize the patient for noncompliance if blood pressure does not improve, or the patient may be bitterly disappointed if careful adherence is not rewarded by a fall in blood pressure. Although we do not want to discourage them from putting forth their best efforts, it is important to be sure that patients understand that the impact of dietary changes on blood pressure cannot be predicted for individuals. (We think it is helpful to point out the many other health advantages associated with the dietary changes they are about to undertake.) Because of these uncertainties, we also advocate caution in placing the "blame" for treatment failure.

Assessment procedures. Although certainly the ideal, comprehensive assessment is simply not practical in most clinics. If cost is not an issue, patient compliance will be. In order to maximize compliance, we try to limit assessments to those we believe are essential. Accordingly, we emphasize self-monitoring of food intake activity for weight reduction and periodic urine sodium analyses for sodium reduction. Figure 7–1 shows the food and activity self-monitoring form we use in our clinic. The form is printed on legal-sized paper and can be folded to easily fit a pocket or handbag. The usefulness of self-monitoring food intake and activity in behavioral weight-control programs can hardly be over-estimated, even though accuracy can be questioned (Dubbert & Brubaker, 1987). Our other routine assessments for weight-reduction patients are weight, height, and skinfold thickness at four sites (triceps, biceps, subscapular, and suprailiac) (Dubbert, in press). We measure height at pretreatment, weight every week, and skinfolds at 3-month intervals.

Assessment of sodium intake is difficult, even with highly motivated subjects (Caggiula, Wing, Nowalk, Milas, Lee, & Langford, 1985; Gillum, Prineas, & Elmer, 1984). One problem is that much of the sodium in many people's diets is in prepared and processed foods, and unless the food is labeled, it may not be possible to determine the actual sodium content. If individuals are accustomed to a high sodium intake, even foods that are extremely high in sodium may not taste salty. Many studies have documented the poor correlation between self-recorded sodium intake and sodium excreted in urine specimens collected during the same time period. Any one single measurement of sodium intake, whether taken from a self-monitoring record or a urine specimen, can be extremely misleading and is simply not very useful for the treatment of an individual patient. Recent studies suggest, however, that by collecting multiple 24-hour specimens, or overnight specimens it is possible to classify patients into low (probably adherent) or high (probably nonadherent) groups with reasonable accuracy (Luft, Fineberg, & Sloan, 1982). Therefore, when possible, we try to collect several urine specimens for each assessment; these are analyzed by the hospital laboratory. However, because collecting these specimens is very inconvenient for most people and because incomplete specimens are useless, we often have to live with missing data.

Fortunately, some new methods of assessing sodium excretion are now being marketed, which may make the assessment of sodium excretion much easier. Early studies indicate the new methods correlate well with 24-hour urine specimens (Luft, Fineberg, & Sloan, 1982; Luft, Sloan, Fineberg, & Free, 1983). These methods involve assessing excretion of chloride (which correlates well with sodium intake) in

Name _____
SS# _____
Address _____
_____
_____ Zip

Phone _____

Jackson VA Medical Center
Heart Health Program

Diet and Exercise
Weekly Record

Goals for this week: _____

Weight Loss _____ pound(s)

Habit Changes: _____
_____
_____

Comments: _____

Date: _____
TIME	FOOD

Date: _____
TIME	FOOD

Date: _____
TIME	FOOD

TIME	ACTIVITY

TIME	ACTIVITY

TIME	ACTIVITY

172

Date: _____
TIME FOOD

Date: _____
TIME FOOD

Date: _____
TIME FOOD

Date: _____
TIME FOOD

TIME ACTIVITY

TIME ACTIVITY

TIME ACTIVITY

TIME ACTIVITY

FIGURE 7-1. Food and Activity Self-Monitoring Form

overnight urine specimens. Collecting an overnight urine specimen is very much easier than collecting all urine for an entire 24-hour period. Preliminary studies suggest these dipstick-type devices (Quantabs, Ames Laboratories) may be simple enough for patients to use in their own homes (Luft et al., 1984). Because the preferred measures may change rapidly as a result of these recent developments, we suggest discussing the best method for assessing changes in sodium intake with patients' referring physicians. It is easiest to leave the collection of urine specimens and interpretation of laboratory results for sodium excretion to the physician's staff; however, you need to know the reliability and validity of the methods used.

Overview of the Program

Table 7–3 shows the major content of each weekly session for the diet-change initiation program. The program consists of two parts or phases, the first emphasizing weight reduction and the second emphasizing sodium reduction. The two parts can be used independently and, in fact, the weight control component was first developed and tested independently with normotensives and hypertensives at Rutgers University (Dubbert & Wilson, 1984). Within each phase, sessions can be repeated if necessary until the content is mastered. Primarily because the results are more evident (and therefore reinforcing to the patient) and because the impact on blood pressure is likely to be more important, we always begin with the weight-reduction segment.

Plan for individualized treatment phase. This program is goal oriented rather than technique oriented. Most behavioral techniques for changing eating habits are presented to patients as optional tools to help them achieve the prescribed dietary goals. In other words, if they can limit food intake without using some of the specific techniques, that is okay. We find that a goal-oriented program, which allows considerable flexibility in decisions about when and how diet changes are accomplished, works well with our population of patients, who are almost all referred rather than volunteers, and often somewhat resistant to the idea of dietary change.

For weight-loss patients, the 10-week program (or 5 weeks if the patient does not need to reduce sodium) is designed as the basis for an extended individualized treatment period. The behavioral obesity research literature indicates clearly that a 10-week program does not produce sufficient momentum to sustain weight loss, but extended treatment can result in weight reductions that compare favorably with

Table 7-3. Weekly Session Content

Part I: Emphasis on Weight Reduction

Session/Week   Content

---

1. Introduction, rationale, expectations for participation. Discuss myths about weight reduction. Practice self-monitoring (retrospective past 24 hours), begin daily food and activity record and daily weighing.
2. Weigh-in, review records. Determine major sources of excess intake, set initial habit change goals.
3. Weigh-in, review records, discuss changes accomplished. Discuss behavior chains. Set new goals.
4. Weigh-in, review records, identify problems. Discuss influence of thoughts and emotions on food intake, and introduce cognitive restructuring techniques. Set new goals, recommend attention to cognitive and emotional factors during the week.
5. Weigh-in, review records, identify problems, Discuss role of increased physical activity in weight reduction. Begin setting food and exercise calorie goals.

Part II: Emphasis on Sodium Reduction

---

6. Weigh-in. Review rationale for sodium reduction. Discuss major sources of sodium in diet. Set goal to eliminate salt at the table and in cooking. Briefly review any weight program problems. Continue monitoring food and activity.
7. Weigh-in. Discuss progress toward last week's goal. Set new goals to eliminate high-sodium snacks and identify substitutes for salted, smoked, and processed meats and cheeses.
8. Weigh-in. Discuss progress toward previous goals. Set new goals: substituting new herbs and spices for high-sodium seasonings and new items for high-sodium condiments.
9. Weigh-in. Discuss progress toward previous goals. New goal: eliminate use of high-sodium canned vegetables and soups and any other prepared foods.
10. Weigh-in. Major progress review, including feedback on urine sodium excretion changes. Assess progress toward caloric- and sodium-reduction goals by comparing this week's food intake to prescribed pattern. Assess progress toward exercise goal.

---

any other nonsurgical intervention (Brownell & Foreyt, 1986). In our current program, the final phase of treatment consists of individualized treatment sessions and is open-ended in length. Treatment sessions in this phase may repeat and expand on the content of the basic program and also need to contain material not included, such as relapse-prevention planning and methods for optimizing social support. In our program, we do not have a standardized approach for dealing with these issues, but rather each therapist designs an individual plan for each patient. While we strongly advocate sessions be held weekly during the initial phase, less frequent sessions (e.g., every other week or even less often if weekly weigh-ins are maintained) can be effective during the individualized treatment phase. We find that many patients become less committed to the program after 4 to 6 months, when they have usually achieved significant weight loss, and in that case we graduate them to a "maintenance" phase with the option of returning to more intensive treatment should they wish to lose more weight or begin to regain. There are many published behavioral-treatment-program manuals with good ideas for weekly assignments dealing with specific problem areas, so we will not provide details here.

PART I: EMPHASIS ON WEIGHT REDUCTION

Week 1

The first session covers a lot of territory. We include here much of the information we try to cover with patients.

Introduction:

You have been told by your physician that losing weight and cutting down on the amount of salt in your diet can help your blood pressure. The dietitian has talked with you about your typical diet, favorite foods, and methods of preparing food, and has worked with you to develop a diet plan that minimizes the changes you have to make. Still, the thought of dieting long enough to lose all that weight and giving up so many foods because they are high in sodium may seem overwhelming. Some people are able to take the diet plan worked out by the dietitian and make the changes fairly quickly. In our experience, those people are unusual and we do not know how long they keep up the diet after they start. Our program is designed for someone like you, who wants to make the changes but doesn't feel totally confident about it, and who would like to take advantage of what psychologists have learned about the best ways to make lasting changes.

This program emphasizes setting goals that are practical and then finding ways to meet those goals. Goals are important. You want to lose weight and may have in mind how many pounds you want to lose. You also have a sodium-intake goal you have been told may benefit your health. If you only think of the final goals, you are likely to be discouraged every time you realize how much effort reaching those goals will require. This program will emphasize goals you can meet in a short time, so you can feel successful every week. That's one of the keys to eventual success.

Although you have two goals, sodium and weight reduction, for the first 5 weeks we will be working primarily on weight reduction. For one thing, it's much easier to measure weight loss than changes in sodium, and by reducing your food intake in order to lose weight you will have made a head start on the sodium reduction.

This weight-loss program is based on energy balance. Think of your body as an engine. Food is the fuel. Eating even a little more than the body needs causes slow weight gain because the body stores the extra fuel as fat. There are two ways to use up the stored fat: (1) cutting back on food (fuel) intake by eating less, and (2) increasing your fuel requirements by increasing your activity. You are going to learn how to regulate your fuel intake and energy output so your body will burn the excess fat while preserving healthy muscle tone. We include a lot of emphasis on physical activity in the program because this helps you feel better and slim down more quickly than you could if you only cut back on what you eat.

This program can help you get better control over your diet. No special diets or pills are used because there aren't any that have been shown to be effective for the long term. You may have been a victim of the "yo-yo syndrome"—gain and lose, gain and lose. Because ths is self-defeating, we will encourage you to make gradual changes in your lifestyle that will allow you to meet your diet goals. You will have to change many eating and activity habits in order to become and stay a thinner person. You learned those habits over many years. You can expect it to take some time for the new behaviors your diet requires to become habits.

Facts and myths about weight loss. We use a little quiz (Table 7–4) as a method of covering some essential physiology and psychology of weight reduction.

You may already know quite a bit about weight control, from your own experience, articles in magazines, talking with friends, and so forth. Even the experts don't agree on everything, but some of the advertisements, books, and articles that get published are not even scientifically accurate. Check your knowledge—try the quiz that follows. Don't be too upset if you don't know the answers—we tried to make the questions interesting so we could discuss some important points.

Beginning self-monitoring. At this point, we take out the forms needed for self-monitoring and begin our instructions for this critical component of the program:

Keeping accurate records of your eating and activity habits is absolutely necessary in this program. In the beginning, we will show you how to use these records to decide what changes are needed in your eating habits. Later the records will help you keep close watch on your own progress. You should expect that this program will take at least 30 minutes of your time each day. Later on, you won't need as much time to keep the records, but you'll be using the time to exercise. If you are not willing to keep the food and activity records, this program will not work for you.

You will be writing down the amounts of all the foods you eat and all the beverages you drink except for plain water. The hardest part about the food records may be estimating how much you ate or drank. It will help a great deal if you measure foods and drinks with a food scale, measuring cup, tablespoon, whatever, for a short time because it is easy to under- or overestimate the amounts. Then you will record the calorie values of the food you ate.

Table 7-4. Do You Know the Facts About Weight Reduction?

(The answers are below.)
T F 1. Dieting success depends mostly on "will power."
T F 2. Even if you stick to your diet, you can't expect to lose weight *every* week.
T F 3. One of the best ways to lose weight and keep it off is to cut out starchy foods such as bread, potatoes, and noodles.
T F 4. Many people find it easier to control how much they eat if they exercise regularly.
T F 5. You can tell how much extra fat is in your body just by weighing.
T F 6. Many people can improve their physical fitness just by walking several times per week.
T F 7. Some foods combine chemically in the body to burn fat and help you lose faster.
T F 8. You can lose weight and still eat most of your favorite foods.
T F 9. If you go off a diet for even one or two days, you'll never be able to get back in control.
T F 10. You'll lose more weight in the long run if you make a big deal out of losing every little pound.

Answers to Quiz
1. FALSE because success in weight control depends on habit change. There is no magical thing called will power, although self-confidence about being able to control eating is important. Set small realistic goals and your success with these will help you develop the confidence you need.
2. TRUE because your body can sometimes store water for a while even though you have burned off fat, making the weight loss uneven. Some weeks you may lose 2 or more pounds but some weeks you may lose nothing.
3. FALSE because those foods are not high in calories by themselves—it's the butter, cream, gravy, and other trimmings that create the problem.
4. TRUE. Scientists aren't sure why, but many obese people do not automatically eat more to make up for calories used up in exercise. It may be that regular exercise makes us more aware of our bodies and less likely to eat foods we know are not healthy.
5. FALSE because the scale can't tell you how much of your body is fat, muscle, and other tissue. Muscle weighs more than the same amount of fat. As you improve your fitness and become more active, you should begin to increase your muscle tissue even as you burn up fat. Although this may mean you won't lose as much weight on the scale, you'll feel better and find it easier to keep your weight off because muscle tissue uses more energy.
6. TRUE because fast walking, for a half hour or more at a time, particularly if you swing your arms, if often sufficient to improve your fitness.
7. FALSE—unfortunately, a calorie in a grapefruit is the same in the body as a calorie in a chocolate cupcake. There are no magic combinations. However, *when* you eat may be important. You may lose weight more easily if you eat 3 meals a day rather than eating the same total amount all in one meal in the evening.
8. TRUE because it's the amount, in calories, that matters. If you can't live without ice cream, you can still lose weight. But you will probably have to eat much less than you would like. Some people prefer not to eat a high-calorie food if they can have only a small amount—that's an individual decision. If you think you need treats now and then, plan for them.
9. FALSE. Going off any program does not doom you to failure, although you may feel that way initially. It's what you do about it that makes the difference. That's why we will work with you until you have built up enough confidence to get back on the program if you have a temporary setback.
10. TRUE because you'll feel better about yourself and the program if you reward yourself for many small successes rather than holding out for the final goal.

We suggest patients buy a calorie-counting book at one of the local book stores, but we also give them a very basic calorie guide to get them started. (See Table 7–5.)

> In order to give us an idea about your typical activity level, you will also be recording all vigorous activity. (We don't require recording routine light activities, because increasing these will have less impact on your weight program.) You will write down each vigorous activity, how long it lasted, and the estimated calorie value. A good way to judge if an activity is vigorous enough to be counted is if it makes you breathe a little harder, increases your heart rate, and/or makes you begin to perspire. If you think an activity was at least in the moderate category, but is not listed on the activity guide (Table 7–6), put it in the category with other activities which seem most similar.
>
> For the first week, you do not have to make any special efforts to reduce your usual calorie intake or try to increase your activity. Instead, eat and exercise (or don't exercise) as usual, and your record will serve as a guide for making changes through the next few weeks. Before you go, we'll start your record for this week.

We then help the patient complete a 24-hour retrospective food and activity calorie record (making a point of telling them it is best to record as soon as possible).

Week 2

Assessment of progress during treatment. Each weekly session begins with a weigh-in and a review of the food and activity records. Patients will often be quite anxious about the weigh-in and eager to talk about the results, but we try not to get caught up in a speculative discussion of the possible reasons for any change (or lack of change). Instead, we use the food and activity data recorded by the patient as the basis for discussion of progress.

Interpreting the food and activity records.

> Now that you have kept careful records of your food intake, we can see which foods contribute the most calories to your diet and how many calories you usually expend through exercise. Recall from last week that goals are important in this program. Specific goals are best. This week, you'll be asked to set specific goals to change one or two eating behaviors in order to reduce your caloric intake. In a couple of weeks you'll also begin to set goals to increase the calories you burn through exercise. It's important to choose positive goals instead of negative ones, such as "I won't eat donuts." Most people find it easier to build positive habits that can replace unhealthy patterns, rather than to simply give up all the old familiar patterns. For example, if you usually eat a snack at coffee-break time, you can set a goal to substitute a piece of fruit rather than giving up your coffee break.

Table 7-5. Food Calorie Guide

MILK GROUP:

1 serving = about 90 calories;
1 cup skim milk or buttermilk,
$\frac{3}{4}$ cup plain low-fat yogurt,
$\frac{1}{2}$ cup lowfat cottage cheese,
$\frac{1}{2}$ cup whole milk.

MEAT/MEAT SUBSTITUTES:

1 portion = about 70 calories;
1 egg,
1 tablespoon peanut butter,
$\frac{1}{3}$ cup lowfat cottage cheese,
$\frac{1}{4}$ cup tuna, lobster, crab, salmon;
5 small scallops, shrimp, oysters, clams (not fried!),
$\frac{1}{2}$ cup cooked dried peas, beans,
8–10 walnuts, pecans, or almonds.

1 portion = about 150 calories;
$\frac{1}{2}$ chicken breast, or leg and thigh, with skin removed,
2 slices roast beef or pot roast, $3 \times 3 \times \frac{1}{4}$ inches, no fat,
$3 \times \frac{1}{2}$ inch hamburger,
2 oz lean lamb or veal.

FATS AND OILS:

1 serving = about 40 calories;
1 teaspoon margarine or butter,
1 teaspoon vegetable oil,
1 teaspoon mayonnaise,
1 teaspoon salad dressing,
1 tablespoon cream.

STARCHY VEGETABLES AND LEGUMES:

1 serving = about 70 calories;
$\frac{1}{3}$ cup corn kernels,
1 small corn on the cob,
$\frac{1}{2}$ cup lima beans,
$\frac{1}{2}$ cup cooked peas, beans, lentils, chickpeas,
1 small 2-inch potato,
$\frac{1}{4}$ cup cooked sweet potato.

BREADS AND CEREALS:

1 serving = about 70 calories;
$\frac{1}{2}$ bagel,
1 slice bread,
one 2 to 3-inch roll,
1 small 2-inch biscuit or muffin,
one $\frac{1}{2}$-inch square cornbread,
$\frac{1}{2}$ English muffin,
$\frac{1}{2}$ hamburger or hot dog bun,
$\frac{1}{2}$ cup bran flakes,
five 2-inch saltines,
$1\frac{1}{2}$ cup popcorn,
$\frac{1}{2}$ cup cooked cereal,

Table 7-5 (*continued*)

BREADS AND CEREALS (*continued*):

¾ cup dry cereal,
½ cup cooked spaghetti, noodles, or macaroni,
¼ cup bread crumbs,
3 tablespoons flour,
2½ tablespoons cornmeal.

LOW-CALORIE VEGETABLES:

1 serving = ½ cup = about 15 calories;
asparagus, green beans, waxed beans, beet greens, broccoli, brussels sprouts, cabbage, cauliflower, celery, collards, cucumber, mushrooms, mustard greens, okra, green and red pepper, radishes, sauerkraut, spinach, summer squash, tomato, tomato juice, turnip greens.

1 serving = 1 cup or more = *eat freely*;
chicory, endive, escarole, lettuce, watercress

MEDIUM-CALORIE VEGETABLES:

1 serving = about 35 calories;
½ cup artichoke,
½ cup beets,
½ cup carrots,
½ cup onions,
¼ cup green peas,
¼ cup pumpkin,
¼ cup winter squash,
½ cup turnips.

FRUITS:

1 serving = about 40 calories;
1 small apple,
⅓ cup apple juice, cider,
2 medium apricots,
½ small banana,
½ cup blackberries,
10 large cherries,
¼ whole cantaloupe,
½ grapefruit,
12 medium grapes,
⅛ whole small honeydew melon,
1 nectarine,
¾ small papaya,
1 medium peach,
1 small pear,
½ cup unsweetened pineapple,
⅓ cup pineapple juice,
2 medium plums,
2 medium prunes,
2 tablespoons raisins,
¼ cup prune juice,
1 cup strawberries,
½ cup raspberries,
1 large tangerine,
1 cup diced watermelon.

Table 7-6. Activity Guide

MODERATELY HARD ACTIVITIES (about 4 calories per minute)
Bicycling 10 to 12 minutes per mile, calisthenics, carpentry work, dancing, garden and
yard work (raking, pushing mower, cutting hedges), golfing (carrying own clubs), house
painting, plastering, scraping paint, mopping, sweeping, scrubbing, table tennis,
volleyball, walking 20 minutes per mile.

HARD ACTIVITIES (about 7 calories per minute)
Vigorous badminton, doubles tennis, basketball, bicycling 6 to 8 minutes per mile, fast
dancing, pick and shovel work, shoveling snow, moderately fast skating, water skiing,
walking 12 minutes per mile, weight training.

VERY HARD ACTIVITIES (about 10 calories per minute)
Boxing, climbing stairs, bicycling, racing, aerobic dancing, judo, running/jogging 6 to 10
minutes per mile, fast skating, cross-country or downhill skiing, squash, racquetball
singles, tennis singles, swimming fast.

This part of the session can take a long time. Interpreting the food
records can be quite difficult if the patient reports eating many "fast" or
processed foods that are not on the food calorie list or if the recording is
vague. It may be necessary to refer patients back to the dietitian for help
in determining the calorie values of food entries, particularly those not
on the exchange list but likely to reappear on future records. We
recommend consulting with a dietitian to get a good up-to-date
calorie-counting guide and also having on hand information about the
caloric content of common fast foods.

After reviewing the records, most patients will have identified a
number of food-choice changes that will be needed to reduce caloric
intake to the prescribed level. We ask them to commit to one (or at most
two) such changes for the next week and record these goals on the new
weekly self-monitoring form. They are also asked to continue recording
time spent in vigorous activities and the corresponding caloric value.
Even though goals are not required at this point in the program, the
reactive effects of self-monitoring often produce an increase in voluntary
activity.

Although sodium reduction is not emphasized during this phase of
the program, patients are likely to reduce their sodium intake
significantly if they avoid processed foods high in sodium. We
specifically caution patients not to use prepared low-calorie foods (such
as Lean Cuisine and Weight Watchers entrees), because these are very
high in sodium content. (In fact, we know of individuals who became
hypertensive while dieting and relying heavily on these products.) It is
best for patients to expect to have to spend more time in food
preparation and meal planning from the very beginning of the diet
rather than to turn to commercially prepared convenience foods high in
sodium. Your consulting dietitian can recommend acceptable "fast"
foods commercially available in your community.

Week 3

The session opens with the weigh-in and progresses immediately to the record review. Patients are asked to comment on their progress toward meeting last week's goal. We then review the food records carefully to determine important remaining high-calorie food choices.

The role of cues in controlling eating behavior. This week's session is designed to teach patients to recognize that internal and external cues may trigger inappropriate and unplanned consumption of high-calorie foods. We present the idea that cues can be powerful determinants of behavior, using examples such as the inviting smells blown out of bakeries to entice customers. Patients are usually able to identify a number of cues that make it more difficult for them to control eating. The next concept we introduce is that of *behavior chains*, with one cue or behavior setting the stage for another, making a chain whose final link is inappropriate eating. Figure 7–2 shows an example. We then have the patient generate several chains, using combinations of internal and external cues.

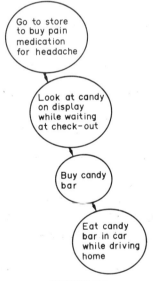

FIGURE 7-2

The important point for this discussion is that some links of the behavior chain are weaker (i.e., easier to control) than others. In the example in Figure 7–2, the person might not have been able to avoid the trip to the drugstore, but he could have looked away or read a magazine to distract himself while waiting to pay for the merchandise. We then ask patients to identify the weak links in the chains they generated

Table 7-7. Suggestions for Changing Food Cues

1. Eliminate all high-calorie "junk" foods from your home. If other family members want them, they must eat them somewhere else.
2. Have prepared vegetables ready for snacks.
3. Replace beverages with diet sodas or mineral water.
4. Put only single servings on the dinner table. If anyone wants seconds, he can go to the stove and serve himself.
5. Weigh or measure the food before you eat it.
6. Use a smaller plate.
7. When at a restaurant, keep the condiments, rolls, and butter off the table, or at least at the other end, out of reach. If others in your party are dieting too, tell the waiter or waitress not to bring these items.
8. Slow down your eating: Put your fork down after every bite.
9. Eat only in the designated dining area.
10. Eat only when sitting down.
11. Don't allow food where eating should not occur (car, desk, bedroom).
12. Don't offer to get food for someone else. Let each adult serve herself. Let someone else serve the children's plates.
13. Eat 3 meals a day, with a large salad or bowl of soup before the main meal.
14. Ask your family and friends not to urge you to eat.
15. Be aware of everything you eat; don't allow distraction by television or by other family members.

earlier. (Patients will often recognize that emotions are an internal cue that links an upsetting event with inappropriate eating; we inform them that this will be the main topic of the next week's session.) For the following week, they are asked to try to recognize chains of events that lead to unplanned inappropriate eating. Patients may be given the stimulus-control suggestions shown in Table 7–7 in written form, or we may suggest pertinent items during the discussion. Finally, with the new information in mind, patients are asked to identify their eating-habit-change goal for the following week and write this on the cover of the self-monitoring form.

Week 4

The first 15 to 20 minutes may be devoted to the weigh-in, review of food records, and discussion of what has been achieved thus far toward reducing total calorie intake. Patients should have made sufficient changes in their eating by this time to begin showing weekly weight loss of about 1 pound per week.

Coping with troublesome thoughts and feelings. During Week 3, we emphasized how cues can affect behavior:

CUE → BEHAVIOR

Much of our routine behavior is made up of habits and behavior chains in which cues lead to behaviors almost automatically. Despite our habits, we are thinking creatures, and many times the way cues affect behavior is through our thoughts:

$$CUE \rightarrow THOUGHT \rightarrow BEHAVIOR$$

Just as habits can be helpful or unhelpful, so thoughts can be (i.e., some thoughts help and some hinder self-control efforts). This session's purpose is to help patients learn how to replace troublesome self-reactions with more appropriate ones. (See Chapter 6 in Mahoney and Mahoney, 1976, as a primary source for this session's material.) Two examples we often use with our patients are:

CUE	THOUGHT	BEHAVIOR
You eat two donuts for breakfast.	Oh, well, I blew it for today . . . might as well chalk up this day for lost.	Eat sweets the rest of day.
Walked 5 miles and only lost 1 pound.	This is torture. I exercise and starve myself and only lose one pound–I'll never be thin.	Stop exercising, watch television.

Different intervening thoughts might lead to quite different behaviors:

You eat two donuts for breakfast.	Wow . . . that used up 500 calories. I can still have a good day.	Eat less the rest of the day.
Walked 5 miles and only lost 1 pound.	It takes time to burn up that fat . . . I didn't gain all my extra weight in one week.	Continue exercising and dieting.

Some patients report eating in response to distressing feelings, such as loneliness, pain, and frustration. Breaking these troublesome links requires recognizing them and then problem solving to identify alternative behaviors. An example:

Feeling frustrated $\rightarrow$ Buy a candy bar and eat it
versus
Feeling frustrated $\rightarrow$ Go for a brisk walk

We reassure patients that this session is only an introduction to the use of these techniques in eating—and exercise-behavior control. In future problem-solving sessions, we will help them apply these to real problems they experience as the weeks go by. As time permits, we help them identify some of their own recent troublesome thoughts and feelings that set the occasion for inappropriate eating.

The session closes with setting one or two habit-change goals for the following week. Changing troublesome thoughts or substituting an alternative to eating as a way of coping with one kind of distressful feelings would be logical choices.

Week 5

Prior to the session, the therapist reviews the activity records from the previous weeks in order to determine the baseline level of vigorous activity. Following the preliminary weigh-in and review of food records, the therapist presents this information to the patient, for example, "According to your records, your average vigorous activity each week consists of walking, house and yard work, and climbing some stairs, for a total of about 300 calories a week." The emphasis in this session is on finding ways to increase average weekly energy expenditure while maintaining the reduced food intake.

Increasing physical activity. Our program recommends brisk walking for most patients as their primary form of exercise. We recommend they set a goal to walk fast, but at a pace that does not leave them breathless, for a minimum of 30 minutes, 5 days each week. Warm-up should consist of slowly increasing the walking speed over the first 5 minutes and cool-down should consist of slowly decreasing the walking speed during the last 5 minutes. We teach patients to check their heart rates, using either the radial or carotid pulse, before and 10 minutes into the exercise period. They are instructed to try to work toward walking at a speed at which their heart rate is in the "target zone" for aerobic training (70% to 80% of age-predicted maximal heart rate). In addition to beginning the regular walking program, we encourage them to continue the same level of vigorous activity in the other forms of exercise they recorded during the past few weeks.

We find that most patients will have achieved fairly good compliance with the recommended level of caloric restriction by the fourth or fifth week. (If not, we continue with the habit-change goals until they are losing weight steadily, even if not in compliance with the original calorie goals). Now, adding an exercise component should significantly increase energy expenditure and may increase the rate of weight loss. Regular exercise of the intensity and frequency we recommend can confer a number of health benefits. (See McArdle, Katch, & Katch, 1981, an excellent exercise physiology reference for the therapist, and Cooper, 1977, a popular book enjoyed by many of our patients).

PART II: EMPHASIS ON SODIUM REDUCTION

Week 6

This week's session begins the second phase of treatment and the beginning of focused effort toward sodium reduction. Current sodium excretion should be assessed at this time and feedback provided to the patient regarding the results. Sodium excretion will be evaluated again at the end of this phase to determine if the food-habit changes have been sufficient to reduce intake to the prescribed 87 mEq level. If patients are adhering to the prescribed caloric-intake goal, they have probably already eliminated or reduced many high-sodium foods, such as potato chips and cheeses. However, total sodium intake may still be too high if they are using salt at the table, food products with added sodium such as canned vegetables, and high-sodium condiments such as pickle relish. This phase of the diet intervention is a step-by-step approach to eliminating remaining sources of excess sodium.

Introduction.

> Your physician has recommended a moderate level of sodium restriction of sodium in your diet because this often helps improve blood pressure control. You have already made a number of changes in your diet and have probably already significantly reduced the amount of sodium you consume. There are so many sources of sodium in most people's diets, though, that we are going to take 5 weeks to eliminate any remaining high-sodium foods and give you a chance to experiment with alternative seasonings. Gradual sodium reduction may be easier for you, too, because you will begin to lose your taste for salt once you reduce your usual intake.
>
> Sodium is one of the minerals that is essential for life. Yet the diets of most Americans contain as much as 10 times as much as the body needs. Most of the time this does not seem to cause any harmful effects, but excessive sodium and water in the body may cause increases in blood pressure or complicate treatment of hypertension with medications. Sodium and salt are not the same. Salt is sodium chloride, which is about one half sodium by weight. Many seasonings, food preservatives, baking powder, and some medications contain high amounts of sodium.
>
> You will have a series of goals for eliminating the high-sodium foods in your diet. This week's goal is to stop using any salt at the table or in cooking. This includes garlic salt and celery salt and high-sodium seasonings such as soy sauce, bouillon, and MSG. But don't just give up the salty seasoning—try some new seasonings instead.

If the patient has not already received some materials with suggestions for seasoning alternatives, we give them the suggestions shown in Table 7–8.

Patients are asked to continue monitoring their food-intake calories and exercise calories each day for the following week.

Week 7

During the record review, it is important to provide praise and encouragement for maintaining the caloric-intake and expenditure goals in addition to meeting the new goals for sodium reduction. At this session, we ask patients to tell us about their reactions to giving up the salt shaker and inquire about any experimentation with alternate

Table 7-8. Sensational Taste Without Sodium: Try These Substitutes

Seasonings	*Use With*
Allspice	Ground meats, stew meats, cookies, fruit
Almond extract	Fruits or baked products
Bay leaves	Meat, poultry, casseroles
Caraway	Salads, noodles, cabbage
Cinnamon	Fruits, especially apples
Curry powder	Meats, especially lamb, chicken
Dill	Eggs, meat, salads, fresh vegetables
Garlic, garlic powder	Meats, mixed with butter
Ginger	Fruits, cookies, oriental dishes
Horseradish	Meats, vegetables
Mace	Desserts
Marjoram	Fruits, green beans, peas
Mustard (dry)	Ground beef, salad dressings
Nutmeg	Desserts, meats, eggs, chicken
Onion	Meats, salads, vegetables, rice, noodles
Oregano	Tomato dishes, meats
Paprika	Meats, fish, noodles
Pepper, black	Meats, vegetables, salads
Poultry seasoning	Chicken, fish
Sage	Meat, green beans
Thyme	Eggs, meats, peas, salads
Vanilla extract	Desserts
Vinegar	Salads, vegetables, marinades

seasonings. (If they have not tried any different seasonings yet, this will be a goal for Week 8.)

This week's food-change goals are to eliminate any remaining high-sodium snack foods and cured meats. Lean ham is not high in calories, but it must be eliminated from the combination weight-and-sodium-reduction diet. The dietitian will have provided the patient with a specific list of foods that must be avoided or eaten in moderation in these categories.

Week 8

The new goals for this week involve eliminating any remaining high-sodium condiments, such as catsup, pickle relish, and prepared mustard. If patients have not already started to experiment with the alternative seasonings, their goal for this week should be to try some of these substitutes. Otherwise, with almost all familiar seasonings eliminated, food will seem bland and tasteless. The dietitian will have given the patient the list of foods to be eliminated.

Week 9

The final high-sodium foods will be eliminated this week. Canned vegetables and soups are typically high in sodium unless they are especially marked "low sodium". Fortunately, low-sodium vegetables and tomato products (including spaghetti sauce) are now beginning to appear on supermarket shelves. These are not highly priced "dietetic" foods, but products with familiar brand names prepared without added salt. We encourage our patients to purchase these if they use canned products. However, preparing fresh vegetables should be encouraged as an alternative, because they may taste better without added seasonings as well as contain additional vitamins and minerals. Frozen vegetables are an acceptable alternative, except for frozen peas and lima beans which pick up sodium during processing. Urine sodium excretion should be measured this week and/or during the following week.

Week 10

The tenth session is the final session of the sodium-reduction phase, but should also be an important progress review for the weight-reduction component of the diet. Accordingly, this session is an important time to review with the patient (a) all the previous weeks' habit change goals, how well they were accomplished, and how well they are being maintained; (b) the typical diet pattern that has emerged and how well it compares to the prescribed model; (c) the total amount of exercise reported each week and whether the goal set at Week 5 is being maintained or exceeded; (d) the total weight loss thus far (at least 5 to 10 pounds would be expected); (e) the present level of sodium excretion and the change in sodium excretion from the initial measure. Finally, this evaluation should provide the rationale and goals for an extended individualized treatment phase, if appropriate.

WHEN TREATMENT FAILS

Experienced clinicians know all too well that the average results reported for behavioral dietary treatment obscure tremendous variability in response. In most programs, some patients lose a significant amount of weight, some lose very little, and some lose nothing or even gain a few pounds. Such variability is one of the more persistent and unsettling findings of research in treatment of obesity, and may well be an indication that some of the critical variables controlling weight loss are still to be identified. There is considerable variability in maintenance too, after weight-reduction programs are completed. At the present time, although we have some interesting leads, and although the evidence shows that patients given behavioral treatment are likely to do better than those who are merely given dietary instructions, it is still not possible to predict in advance if a given individual will succeed (Dubbert & Wilson, 1983).

In an earlier section, we discussed the importance of cautioning patients that blood-pressure changes may not occur despite excellent dietary adherence. Here we would like to caution therapists to be prepared to help patients make appropriate attributions if they fail to achieve significant weight loss and/or sodium reduction. If the treatment situation permits, more specific assessments may uncover the adherence failures. We have found, however, that failures of adherence are typically accompanied by failures of self-monitoring, so it is often difficult to determine what went wrong. Family/spouse involvement may be helpful in some cases. Other patients will exert more effort after a return to the referring physician and reemphasis on the possible benefits of dietary change. When none of the apparent interventions succeeds, however, we are prepared to try to help the patient view the failure as specific to this particular time and situation rather than as a characterological defect. We always try to leuve the door open for the patients to try diet interventions again when the situation seems more favorable.

Chapter 8

Improving Medication Compliance

Estimates of the extent of noncompliance vary with the type of health problem and nature of the behavior being evaluated (taking medications, following a diet, keeping a scheduled appointment); however, data from a number of studies indicate that more than 50% of all patients can be expected to fail to follow through exactly with medical advice (Dunbar & Stunkard, 1979). Noncompliance appears to be even more of a problem with asymptomatic chronic conditions such as hypertension. Studies show that up to 50% of hypertensive patients fail to follow through on referral advice, over 50% of those who begin treatment drop out within the first year, and only about two thirds of those who stay in treatment take enough of their prescribed medication to achieve good blood pressure control (National Heart, Lung and Blood Institute [NHLBI] Working Group, 1982).

The past two decades have seen a growing recognition of the significance of noncompliance in many areas of medical practice and an ever-increasing literature devoted to studies of compliance behavior (Kolton & Stone, 1986). Although we must direct interested readers to other sources for more extensive and critical reviews; e.g., see Haynes, Taylor, & Sackett, 1979, we thought it important to include in this chapter some discussion of the implications of noncompliance with hypertension drug-treatment regimens as well as methods for detecting and intervening in compliance failure.

DEFINING THE PROBLEM

Compliance is typically defined as the extent to which a person's behavior conforms with the advice of the health care provider (Haynes, 1979). However, some providers and patient advocates take issue with the use of this terminology because, to them, it implies the blame for the problem should be attributed the individual patient. The term *adherence* has been used more frequently in recent literature because it connotes a more democratic, cooperative relationship; a few writers have advocated the use of the term *concordance* rather than *compliance* for the same reason. In our own work, we use the terms compliance and adherence interchangeably and without implying an inequitable distribution of responsibility between provider and patient. Although the major focus of this chapter will be on the patient who fails to take medication as prescribed, it is important to remember that the noncompliance of health care providers to recommended protocols also contributes (to an unknown extent) to treatment failure.

EFFECTS OF NONCOMPLIANCE

The clinical trials of the past two decades have convincingly demonstrated the benefits of drug treatment in all but the mildest blood-pressure elevations. Patients with moderate and severe hypertension can hope to live longer and with less likelihood of complications of high blood pressure if adequately medicated (See Chapter 1). It is certainly discouraging to health care providers that so many hypertensive patients fail to benefit from treatment regimens because of noncompliance, and noncompliance can have other important negative outcomes as well. Failure to follow prescribed therapy may involve the patient in unnecessary diagnostic and treatment procedures, it negatively influences patients' views about services received, and noncooperation makes it difficult to accurately assess the quality of care provided (Becker, 1985).

In most cases, patients will experience no immediate obvious consequences of a variety of patterns of noncompliance (e.g., occasionally forgetting a single dose; consistently taking less than the prescribed amount; omitting medications for days or weeks at a time due to drinking episodes, preoccupation, or short supply). However, with some medications (i.e., short-acting beta-blockers or centrally acting sympathetic agonists), even short-term nonadherence can be dangerous. After chronic therapy with beta-blockers, sudden withdrawal can unmask coronary heart disease, resulting in the emergence of angina or even a myocardial infarct. Rapid withdrawal of the centrally acting sympathetic agonists, particularly clonidine, has been associated with rapid rebound to dangerous levels of high blood pressure.

DETECTING NONCOMPLIANCE

Most providers recognize that noncompliance is one of the major reasons that so many hypertensives remain uncontrolled (Breckenridge, 1983). Measurement of adherence, however, remains a major problem in research and clinical settings. To date, no method has yet achieved the status of the "gold standard" for detection of noncompliance, but there is sufficient evidence to suggest that some methods are more useful than others.

1. *Monitoring attendance.* Although many patients who remain in treatment fail to take adequate medication, noting when patients fail to return for appointments is critical for early detection of potential drop-outs (NHLBI Working Group, 1982).

2. *Monitoring treatment outcome and drug side effects.* A number of studies have shown that compliance and treatment outcome are not highly correlated in clinical populations. When blood pressure control alone is used to identify patients as noncompliant, a large proportion are misclassified. In a study with 245 men, for example, Haynes and his colleagues (Haynes, Taylor, Sackett, Gibson, Bernholz, & Mukherjee, 1980) found that only 67% of patients with controlled blood pressures were compliant by pill count, while 46% of those whose blood pressures remained elevated were compliant. Craig (1985) also found that using uncontrolled blood-pressure readings alone as a measure of compliance would have mislabeled 20% of her patients as noncompliant. Inadequate therapy, overmedication, and failure of individuals to respond to established treatment regimens are some of the reasons for the lack of correspondence between compliance and outcome.

    Breckenridge (1983) believes that the presence of side effects, or pharmacological effects of the prescribed drugs, is more useful than blood pressure control. For example, patients who are taking beta-blocker drugs would be expected to have exercise heart rates less than 100 beats per minute; patients taking clonidine typically complain of having a dry mouth. Failure to observe these side effects in a patient with poorly controlled blood pressure would be suggestive of noncompliance.

3. *Pill counts and prescription refills.* Because this methodology is objective and quantitative, pill counts are used in most compliance research and under carefully controlled circumstances can serve as the standard by which other measures can be evaluated. Pill counts can be relatively reliable if performed unannounced, at the patient's home, and the exact date the patient started using the medication is known. Clinic pill counts are often not very useful because

noncompliant patients may forget to bring their pills or fail to keep their scheduled appointments (NHLBI Working Group, 1982; Haynes et al., 1980). In addition, it cannot be assumed that pills removed from the bottle were ingested by the patient; some patients throw out extra medications when they realize pills are being counted and others share their drugs with family members.

Checking prescription refills is a related method of assessing compliance. Providers in the Jackson VAMC Hypertension Clinic use prescription-refill information supplied by the outpatient pharmacy to identify patients who may not be using medications as prescribed. Patients who have not requested refills at the expected rate between appointments are questioned more carefully about their medication compliance.

4. *Blood and urine analyses.* Body-fluid analyses that monitor levels of drugs, drug metabolities, or markers introduced into medication tablets have been helpful in some areas of medical practice, but have remained of limited use in the treatment of hypertension (Dubbert, King, Rapp, Brief, Martin, & Lake, 1985). Haynes and his colleagues (1980) found that serum potassium, serum urate and urinary chlorthalidone and hydrochlorothiazide assessments were not as useful as patient interviews in classifying compliant and noncompliant patients. There are a number of potential problems with using body-fluid measures. Haynes et al. (1980), for example, found that some patients who were taking inadequate doses of diuretics nevertheless tested positive for the presence of the drug in the urine. Variations in drug absorption and metabolism between patients also limit the accuracy of monitoring both the drugs and chemical markers (Morisky, 1986). Gordis (1979) provides an excellent review of these issues.

5. *Patient interviews.* Several investigators have found that, despite a tendency for overestimation when compared with pill-count compliance, patient self-report is the best single method of compliance assessment (NHLBI, 1982). In studies with hypertensives, Haynes et al. (1980) found that 90% of the patients who admitted noncompliance were found to be noncompliant by pill count. Craig (1985) also found the interview to be the most sensitive measure, with 100% of patients who admitted noncompliance found to be noncompliant by urine assay. In both these studies, 50% to 60% of subjects who reported compliance were found to be noncompliant, resulting in correct overall classification of 75% to 85% by the self-report method. Combinations of self-report, blood, and urine analysis did not improve accuracy of identifying noncompliant patients in Haynes' study. Because some studies indicate that

patients who admit their noncompliance are the most likely to respond to interventions, busy practitioners can reasonably hope to identify about half of the patients who would best respond to compliance interventions by simply asking them in a nonthreatening way if they are having trouble taking their medications (Morisky, 1986; Sackett, 1979).

STRATEGIES FOR IMPROVING COMPLIANCE

A number of methods for improving patient compliance have been advocated, many of them consistent with behavioral and self-regulation models of compliance behavior (NHLBI Working Group, 1982; Peck & King, 1982). A small number of controlled studies have now demonstrated the effectiveness of some of these strategies for improving compliance (Epstein & Cluss, 1982). We review here those we have found most helpful and/or have received the most empirical support thus far.

1. *Identify patients at greatest risk.* If reliable risk factors for noncompliance could be identified, expensive and intrusive detection methods could then be reserved for the patients at highest risk. Recent attempts to identify correlates of compliance in hypertensives suggest that certain patient or regimen characteristics may be associated with increased risk. Several researchers, for example, have found that multiple-dose regimens are associated with poorer compliance (Widmer, Cadoret, & Troughton, 1983; Watts, 1981; Wagner, Truesdale, & Warner, 1981). Age, sex, and race have been predictors of noncompliance in some but not all studies: for example, increased drop-out rates for males as compared with females (DeGoulet et al., 1983), and better appointment and medication compliance for younger as compared with older patients (DeGoulet et al., 1983; Nelson, Stason, Neutra, Solomon, & McArdle, 1978). However, demographic characteristics did not correlate with compliance in a North Carolina survey including many rural blacks and whites (Wagner et al., 1981). Finally, lack of social support has been associated with poor compliance in several studies (James et al., 1984; Nelson et al., 1978; Williams et al., 1985).

2. *Make the regimen as simple as possible.* This follows from the observations in several studies (Wagner et al., 1981; Watts, 1981; Widmer et al., 1983) that patients on multiple-dose regimens are more likely to admit missing doses and show poor blood pressure control. Drug companies have taken note of these findings and it is

now no longer necessary for many hypertensives to take medications several times a day. Simplifying the regimen also means avoiding unnecessary prescriptions (e.g., no potassium supplements unless a significant deficiency exists).

3. *Tailor the treatment program to the patient's lifestyle.* Although there is little empirical evidence to demonstrate the effectiveness of tailoring as a single intervention strategy (Epstein & Cluss, 1982), we would expect that compliance should be improved when treatment regimens minimize the changes required in patients' lifestyles and link new behaviors to established habits (Dunbar & Stunkard, 1979). Haynes and his colleagues (Haynes et al., 1976) included tailoring as part of a package of interventions that significantly improved compliance in a group of Canadian steelworkers. Patients were interviewed to determine any daily habits or rituals and, whenever possible, medications were scheduled to be taken immediately before the habit or ritual was executed.

4. *Arrange cues or prompts* that can help remind patients and health care providers to follow through with prescribed regimens. Haynes et al. (1976) advised patients to place their medications in close proximity to daily habits or rituals as part of the tailoring strategy. In our own work (Dubbert, Martin, & Cushman, 1985), we have found that compliant patients often report using self-generated prompting strategies such as keeping the medication bottle on the table by the toaster, near shaving supplies, or even in a shoe! Although special medication packaging, which might serve a cueing function, has not yet been shown to improve compliance in hypertensives (Eshelman & Fitzloff, 1976), written treatment instructions, personal blood-pressure follow-up cards, and invitations for new check-ups resulted in a reduced drop-out rate for prompted patients when compared with controls (Takala, Niemela, Rosti, & Sievers, 1979). A simple appointment-reminder system, which also employs the strategy of having the patient make a written commitment to return, has been suggested by Frank Masur (personal communication, April 15, 1985). Patients are given a postcard before leaving the office and requested to fill out their name, address, the follow-up appointment date, the provider's name, and the reason for the follow-up visit. The postcard is then placed in a clinic file divided by months. At the first of the month, the entire month's cards are sent out to serve as reminders to the patients to keep their appointments.

5. *Set up a behavioral contract.* Dunbar, Marshall, and Hovell (1979) have identified several advantages in behavioral contracting to improve compliance: (a) devising a contract involves patients in their treatment planning; (b) a written contract outlines expected

behaviors, thus providing a reference in case details are forgotten; (c) a contract brings about a formal commitment from the patient; and (d) a contract specifies incentives for treatment adherence. Swain and Steckel (1981) used behavioral contracting to improve compliance with hypertensives drawn from two medical center clinics. In this study, hypertensives contracted with their nurse to engage in behaviors related to a variety of hypertension-related goals, including keeping clinic appointments, losing weight, recording food intake, recording daily blood pressures, and taking and recording medications (Steckel & Swain, 1977). On average, the behavioral-contract patients showed improved blood pressure control as compared with patients who received an educational intervention or routine clinic care. Behavioral contracting was also a component of the successful program evaluated by Haynes (Haynes et al., 1976), in which patients could earn their own blood-pressure-monitoring equipment if they showed progressive improvements in blood pressure control.

6. *Increase patient involvement through self-management strategies.* Although simple educational strategies appear to be ineffective because they result in improvements in knowledge without changing compliance (Sackett et al., 1975; Swain & Steckel, 1981), more complex educational and self-management programs have produced very encouraging results. For example, Zismer and colleagues (Zismer, Gillum, Johnson, Becerra, & Johnson, 1982) reported significant improvements in diastolic blood pressure for hypertensives who were randomized to an educational program emphasizing pill taking, appointment keeping, and reduced sodium intake. Their educational sessions included goal-setting and self-appraisal of progress with active patient participation. Levine and others (Levine, Green, Deeds, Chwalo, Russell, & Finlay, 1979) also evaluated a comprehensive educational program including three levels of intervention: (1) an exit interview, (2) a home visit, and (3) small group meetings. The exit interview was designed to check patients' understanding of their regimen and tailor it to their individual schedule; the home visit reinforced the exit interview and included a significant other adult in an attempt to increase family/peer support for compliance; and the small group sessions included role play and group problem solving. The combination of all three interventions was most effective in improving blood pressure control, but combination of any two also had some positive effect. In the initial evaluation, the exit interview alone did not improve control over that observed in control patients, but a 5-year follow-up showed a positive effect of having participated in any one or more

components of the educational program. Over time, the experimental patients showed superior appointment keeping, weight control, and blood pressure control (Morisky, Levine, Green, Shapiro, Russell, & Smith, 1983). Notably, the all-cause mortality was 57.3% less and hypertension-related mortality was 53.2% less for experimental patients.

Home blood pressure monitoring failed to improve blood pressure control when used as a single strategy (Carnahan & Nugent, 1975), but Haynes and his co-investigators found a combination of self-monitoring, increased therapist supervision, and contracting increased compliance in patients whose previous nonadherence was well documented (Haynes et al., 1976). Six months later, patients who received the experimental program had improved compliance by 21%, while compliance in the control group had decreased 1.5%. Compliance was measured rigorously by unobtrusive, unannounced pill counts. Finally, Nessman, Carnahan, and Nugent (1980) were able to achieve successful outcomes in previously nonadherent patients through a combination of self-management (home blood pressure monitoring and selection of drugs by patients themselves) and group therapy. After 8 weekly meetings, experimental patients had lower diastolic blood pressures, better pill counts, and better clinic attendance.

7. *Mobilize social support resources.* Social-learning theory suggests a number of ways in which social support could affect compliance. Family members, friends, co-workers and fellow patients may enhance antecedent, consequent, and cognitive control over critical behaviors in the prescribed regimen. Recent studies indicate that a variety of social-support interventions can improve adherence to hypertension drug-treatment regimens. The second and third components of the successful three-stage program described earlier (Levine et al., 1979; Morisky et al., 1983) consisted of a home visit involving a family member or significant other and small group sessions. Nessman et al. (1980) implemented a successful self-management program in a group-treatment format and observed that, over the course of treatment, patient-to-patient interactions increased, while staff-to-patient-initiated communications decreased.

Perhaps the most widely applied social-support strategy to date is the development of programs to treat hypertensives at the worksite. Although an early attempt to improve compliance by providing treatment at the worksite failed (Sackett et al., 1975), several controlled evaluations have now shown that such programs can substantially improve blood pressure control among hypertensive employees (e.g., Alderman & Schoenbaum, 1975; Foote & Erfurt, 1983). However, Foote and Erfurt's (1983) results suggest that worksite screening and referral without additional intervention may increase the number of employees under treatment without producing any long-term improvements in blood pressure control. In contrast, more costly and labor-intensive interventions can result in good control for the majority of employees served by the program. These investigators concluded that the success of worksite interventions can be attributed to three factors that have also been shown to be important in nonworksite programs: aggressive follow-up, provision of information, and positive feedback and support.

Chapter 9

Putting It All Together

High blood pressure, or hypertension, is clearly associated with certain patterns of unhealthy behavior or lifestyle in a considerable proportion of the many who develop the disease. Though hypertension may not be directly produced by these behavioral risk factors, it is almost certainly complicated by their presence. As noted in the previous chapters, overweight, stress, poor diet and physical inactivity have each been implicated in the development of high blood pressure. Additionally, these unhealthy patterns of behavior may serve independently or in combination to retard blood-pressure lowering from pharmacologic therapy as well as to increase absolute blood pressure levels. Finally, recent data also suggest that those with high normal blood pressure (i.e., 85 to 89 mm Hg. diastolic) may be at special risk to develop hypertension eventually if their lifestyle habits are poor (e.g., overweight, sedentary Type A).

At minimum, these unhealthy lifestyles must be effectively modified in order to avoid the necessity of overmedicating the individual. That is, hypertensives who are overweight, sedentary, have a high-sodium diet, and/or who cope with stress poorly, are more likely to require significantly higher doses of antihypertensive agents to overcome the drug-canceling/blood-pressure-elevating effects of their unhealthy behavior. On the other hand, a number of hypertensives may not need medication if they will control their weight, diet, exercise and stress/coping (remember that the majority of the approximately 35 to 50 million Americans with high blood pressure are in the mild range of 90 to 104 mm Hg, diastolic). The behavioral research data on non-pharmacologic treatment of hypertension summarized and illustrated in the previous chapters certainly lend support to this notion. Hence, any medication at all in at least some patients may be considered an unnecessary overdose.

Especially in those who need to be medicated, the coexistence of blood-pressure-elevating health habits will necessitate higher than normal doses of antihypertensive medications. This drug "overtreatment" might subsequently produce toxic side effects, a common occurrence in medicated hypertensives, followed by significant decrements in quality of life (e.g., impotence) and, ultimately, medication noncompliance. The latter concern of medication noncompliance is a particularly common and vexing problem in hypertensive patients. In fact, approximately one third to one half of all treated hypertensives will fail to adhere well enough to their medication regimen to significantly lower their blood pressure over the long term (Haynes, 1979).

Thus far we have focused on stress reduction, diet, and exercise individually. It may be, however, that the sole control of weight, diet, stress or physical activity is insufficient to minimize or eliminate the need for medication in those who have more than one of these risk factors. The changes in that behavioral area which would be required to sufficiently lower blood pressure may be far too difficult to achieve through a single behavioral intervention (e.g., losing 75 pounds *or* severely restricting sodium, alcohol, and cholesterol intake, *or* practicing relaxation three or four times daily, *or* exercising seven days a week for 2 hours at a time). This is particularly evident in the many hypertensives who come to us with clusters of unhealthy "hypertensive behaviors". For example, individuals who are overweight are likely to be sedentary, and vice versa, and have an unhealthy diet and poor stress coping (some have called this the American lifestyle; Farquhar, 1979).

Independent of whether multiple behavioral areas must be targeted for an adequate blood-pressure result is the desire of patients to change in more than one area of their lifestyle. For example, many of our patients were not satisfied with stopping after changing just one behavior, and would often request our help in a variety of areas such as exercise, smoking cessation, and weight reduction.

Clinicians should not underestimate the value of "striking while the iron is hot" and capitalizing on this unique window of opportunity for bringing several problem health behaviors under control within the same therapeutic context and time frame. Patients have echoed such statements as: "Well, I'm going to all the trouble of changing this, and I've got these experts who are willing to help me with the others . . . why not get it all done now!" We would certainly encourage professionals to consider the benefits of this multiphasic approach, while at the same time carefully weighing the potential benefits against the possible risks of therapeutic overload leading to compliance/ adherence problems and subsequent program failure or drop-out.

Thus, in the *likely* event of multiple hypertensive behaviors in the same patient, the health care professional—in conjunction with the patient, and perhaps the patient's family—must decide not only whether to medicate or treat behaviorally, or both, but also what order or combinations of treatments to implement. In this chapter we will discuss the use of multiple behavioral treatment of the high-blood-pressure patient.

COMBINED BEHAVIORAL TREATMENT IN HYPERTENSION

As mentioned in the previous chapter, we have noticed that even some formerly noncompliant and poorly compliant medicated patients who, following careful behavioral training, adhere quite well to the seemingly more complex behavioral programs of weight reduction/diet, stress management, and exercise training. This may be due in part to both the immediate and long-term positive side effects of these lifestyle interventions, as contrasted with the often immediate negative consequences of many medication regimens. When implemented properly (i.e., gradual shaping, using positive reinforcement contingencies) these behavioral regimens can become highly rewarding activities that serve to make the person feel and (in the cases of diet and exercise) look better as well as become healthier. We have also found that patients frequently state a desire to do whatever is necessary to minimize drug side effects as well as their "sick-role" dependence on medication. In fact, recent studies have suggested that placing hypertensives on lifetime medication regimens may significantly impinge upon quality of life and self-attributions of health and sickness (Hovell, 1986).

Ordering Intervention

Once the decision to attempt multiple behavioral interventions has been made, the question of ordering interventions arises. Generally we recommend that the life style-change programs be applied successively rather than concurrently. Though there are very little data on whether it is more effective to combine interventions from the start or to implement them individually, it is our strong belief that patients can be easily overloaded with regimens and it is desirable to avoid complex regimens that have been associated with poor compliance.

We suggest that the simpler the program is at first, the better. Patients should gradually be shaped toward incorporation of all the health-behavior changes desired and required to control blood pressure and improve health (the latter a motive that patients may acquire as they begin to become more healthy and expand their goal from mere control of blood pressure to optimal health). We do not recommend, however, adding a new behavioral regimen until home maintenance has been demonstrated to the satisfaction of the therapist.

In a few cases, individual patients may desire to make several changes at once. They may even make them without consulting with you, so be sure to track collateral behaviors as well. We usually do not require patients to stop these "add-on" programs (for example, changing their diet when on an exercise program), but we caution them against taking on too much at once. This is not to say that patients might not experience a sudden "conversion" to health, and successfully change several unhealthy habits. In this case, caution the patient, and stand ready to intervene and simplify the regimen at the first sign of faltering. Otherwise, lots of encouragement from the therapist, along with frequent contact and family involvement in their program, can be most important in these cases.

We often question patients, as part of our assessment, regarding their preference as to which behavior they would like to target first. Not surprisingly, weight reduction and stress management are often mentioned first. Weight modification is an excellent beginning area in which to intervene, especially if the patient is clearly overweight/overfat, and is highly motivated to lose weight. The advantages of starting with *weight reduction* are that the data supporting its efficacy and potency in lowering blood pressure is probably the strongest. We know that even a weight loss as little as 7 pounds may be sufficient to "normalize" blood pressure in milder hypertensives.

In addition to the fact that it is often the first choice in the many patients who want to improve their physical appearance as well as control blood pressure, weight reduction is also more accepted by the medical community as an important and viable therapeutic goal in the management of their hypertensives. Among the disadvantages of starting with weight reduction, or any dietary intervention for that matter, are that it may be the most difficult to achieve, it requires a more complex cognitive and behavioral regimen than exercise and stress management, and, perhaps most importantly, it generally involves aversive contingencies and consequences (e.g., feeling hungry, resisting delicious foods, and eating less tasty foods in lower quantities). Also, the regimen will usually be complicated because most of the better weight-modification programs involve some form of exercise and, possibly, stress management. Thus, the advantages of starting with weight reduction must be weighed carefully (no pun intended) against some of these important considerations.

On the other hand, both *exercise* and *stress management* can be implemented by themselves, and probably within the context of a less complex or problematic regimen than required for weight/diet change. Both have (or should have) positive consequences (feeling relaxed and calm; feeling invigorated and fit), though exercise is frequently misapplied to a painful level. Obviously, in individuals who are not overweight, dietary interventions may not be appropriate initially. We do caution professionals to be sure to measure body fat as well as weight, because a thin-appearing person may have considerable body fat (though hidden within a seemingly trim body frame) that might contribute significantly to elevated blood pressure. Relaxation training is probably the most parsimonious behavioral treatment and might be an excellent first intervention, especially in hypertensives with particularly high stress levels and/or poor stress coping skills. (It should be remembered, however, that our own data suggest a preference for thermal biofeedback over relaxation.) A therapist might want to begin with a several-week period of relaxation training, and then add exercise.

Careful matching of the history, needs, and desires of the hypertensive with the capabilities of the behavioral regimens should help ensure the effective acquisition and maintenance of the health-behavior change. For example, an individual who has frequently failed to lose weight, or is chronically dieting, might be steered toward exercise or relaxation at first. We sometimes have offered the more desired treatment, one that we feel is too complex to begin with, contingent upon completing so many weeks of a lower rated, but more probably successful health-behavior-change program. Because exercise is often done in enjoyable social contexts, as opposed to solitary relaxation and dieting, we particularly recommend exercise for those hypertensives who are more socially outgoing and/or who seem to require or do better with high levels of social support and reinforcement. Further, if the patient has trouble with mood (i.e., depression) rather than anxiety, we may want to steer them initially to exercise, where they should experience immediate positive consequences in several areas of their life. Especially for medicated patients, when used in conjunction with medications, exercise may also help to minimize the fatigue and depression that accompany certain antihypertensive drug regimens.

MEDICATIONS AND LIFESTYLE CHANGE COMBINED

Some recent data from the Hypertension Prevention and DISH Trials suggest that we may be able to prevent hypertension in some patients through early behavioral interventions, or to control elevated blood pressure rapidly with pharmacotherapy and maintain normotensive levels using behavioral procedures after medications are faded out. (Schlundt & Langford, 1985). In any event, we recommend conferring carefully with the patients' physician or with medical consultants regarding the combination of medication and lifestyle change. We generally suggest, for those hypertensives with blood pressures stabilized between 90 and 104 mm Hg DBP that a trial of approximately 12 weeks of either exercise, diet/weight modification, or stress management be attempted along with their present medication dose. This is probably the safest and most conservative approach. The advantages are that it continues patients on their normal prophylactic drug dose, and does not require quick behavioral results or a physician completely sympathetic to lifestyle approaches to controlling blood pressure. On the disadvantage side, the medications may actually slow the blood-pressure-lowering effect of exercise (data on this is equivocal, because with some drugs, it may actually accelerate the BP drop) or other behavioral interventions, and the patient needs to attend to two different classes of prescribed regimens, a complexity that may be problematic in terms of compliance.

An additional advantage of combined pharmacotherapy and behavioral interventions in hypertension treatment is that aggressive application of one may allow for subsequent minimal use of the other in the long-term management of the disease. In fact, some studies and programs have indicated that the longer an individual with high blood pressure maintains blood pressure control through medication, the longer it may take for blood pressures to return to hypertensive levels. This may also be true for primary nonpharmacological intervention. For example, this phenomenon has been observed in both ours and others' programs (e.g., Langford et al., 1985), although additional research is needed before the validity and reliability of this can be established. Nevertheless, it may be that certain patients who have had their blood pressures controlled for an extended period of time by pharmacotherapy, in whom medications are faded out, may be effectively maintained on behavioral-health changes of the type we have been discussing here.

Clearly, there would appear to be many ways in which a hypertensive with multiple risk factors can be managed using drug and nondrug avenues of treatment. To better illustrate how this might be put together clinically the following case study is offered:

CASE STUDY
Joe M was referred to the Behavioral Medicine Clinic by his physician, a family practitioner. Joe was reasonably well controlled on a low dose of diuretic and sympathetic-dampening beta-blocker drugs: His blood pressure was relatively stable around 130/92 mm Hg,

reduced over a period of 6 months from his baseline levels of 141/101 mm Hg. Despite these positive results, both Joe and his physician were uncomfortable because he was about 25 pounds overweight, ate a diet high in sodium and fat, smoked one pack of cigarettes per day, exercised only once per week (tennis doubles), and he reported high levels of stress in his job as a stockbroker in a large city. After careful baseline assessment on each of these behavioral risk factors and of his blood pressure, the therapist held a counseling session with Joe to determine where to begin.

His strong preference was to lower his stress level or to learn to cope better with the stress (he also suffered from what appeared to be mostly tension headaches). Secondarily, he wanted to lose some weight, but he dreaded giving up favorite foods (his wife was a great cook, he explained, and both of them liked to eat). He refused to stop smoking, even when the risks of malignant hypertension and acceleration of coronary heart disease were detailed for him. Diet and exercise were not quite that "hands-off," but were not high on his "motivation list". The problem for the clinician at this point was whether he should (a) make the stress management contingent upon targeting one of the other critical, but lower probability (for change) behaviors, such as diet/weight, and thus risk early drop-out, or (b) provide alleviating stress management (relaxation) immediately, followed by attempts to modify the remaining risk behaviors. The therapist wisely chose (b), hoping to induce further attempts at lifestyle change once Joe has confidently attributed his success in managing stress to his own abilities, motivation and efforts. Though Joe is only asked to work on his stress levels, the therapist also includes in the initial phase daily home self-monitoring of blood pressure, stress levels, headaches, weight and exercise.

Joe is then asked to sign a written agreement/contract (co-signed by his wife) stating that he will (a) attend weekly sessions for 10 weeks, (b) complete his home relaxation twice very day during the time, and (c) keep daily self-monitoring records of the various risk behaviors/levels. In addition, he agrees to begin working on a second risk behavior of his choosing (i.e., diet, exercise or smoking) by the fifth week. The wife agrees to serve as informant, and to provide reinforcement for compliance (back rubs, special gifts, etc.).

Joe is then given ordered and marked audiotapes (some with embedded tones or code words) of his first (live) relaxation session and asked to practice twice daily and record the word or number of tones, if any, that were on that tape to assess compliance (cf. Martin et al., 1981).

In the fifth week, Joe chooses to add diet. His wife (who is also overweight and wants to lose) is included in diet/weight modification sessions. An additional contract is signed, with deposit, for the amount of weight loss and monitoring of weight and calorie/nutritional intake. Joe and wife are placed on a lower fat diet designed to moderately restrict overall caloric (1500 Kcal/day) and sodium (80 mEq) intake. Relaxation practice is also continued in the home, although sessions are devoted to diet change by Week 5.

By the eighth week, blood pressure had fallen to 125/88 mm Hg, headaches and overall stress levels moderated significantly, and Joe and his wife had lost 7 and 5 pounds, respectively. One week before the end of the contract, Joe was encouraged not to stop now, but to go on and tackle another negative health behavior. Exercise was suggested, since it dovetailed so nicely with weight management, and it was explained that exercise may be essential to maintain the weight loss. Joe agreed, and signed an additional 8-week contract. The contract specified that he would continue to monitor and engage in relaxation, diet/weight control, and exercise.

Prior to beginning exercising, Joe was first referred to a special rehabilitative-medicine facility and was given a full medical workup, including a maximal-graded exercise test. An exercise prescription was provided, and Joe was enrolled in a 3-day-per-week aerobic exercise program. He continued to attend the weekly health-behavior-change sessions, and brought self-monitoring records of his program and home-exercise activity to each session for review and adherence counseling. His wife was encouraged to exercise in the home with him, and each worked gradually to the level of 30 minutes walking per day. Both were provided with pedometers and asked to graph their daily mileage.

At the conclusion of this next 8-week period, both Joe and his wife had lost more than 10 pounds, their sodium and fat intake was significantly less (Mrs. M was cooking using the American Heart Association cookbook), he was faithfully practicing relaxation at least once per day without a tape, both were exercising (brisk walking) enjoyably for approximately 30 to 45 minutes per day at 70% of their capacity (RPE: 12–13), and, best of all, Joe's blood pressure fell during this period to the point (121/82 mm Hg) whereby his physician decided to slowly begin the fading of antihypertensive medications. While the physician carefully monitored Joe's blood pressure at regular medical visits, we carefully monitored and consequated adherence to the behavioral program in monthly visits for a year, and then 3-month follow-up appointments.

Finally, we recommended strongly that Joe seek treatment for his smoking. Given his success in modifying diet, stress and exercise, Joe felt confident enough to accept this challenge, and he was referred (though still followed by us) for aggressive treatment for his smoking.

This case study has illustrated the nondrug management of a medicated hypertensive with multiple behavioral risk factors for high blood pressure and cardiovascular disease. The following section will turn to the early intervention of nonmedicated and *prehypertensives*.

PREVENTION AND EARLY BEHAVIORAL INTERVENTION

Several bodies of evidence, such as the HDFP study (HDFP Cooperative Group, 1976, 1979a, 1979b, 1982a, 1982b), would suggest the importance of aggressively treating even mild hypertension (i.e., DBP = 90 mm Hg.). Also, high-normal blood pressure of 85 to

89 mm Hg DBP appears to be a risk factor for the development of hypertension. Behavioral interventions thus may hold special promise with these two groups of at-risk individuals. These potentially low-cost, and highly effective nonpharmacological approaches to blood pressure control are particularly appropriate first defenses in these cases: Hypertensives may first receive behavioral treatment while maintaining the program on their own, whereas high normals could initiate and continue their behavioral health program with a minimum of education and guidance.

Although some in the medical community wait for blood pressure to reach 95 or 100 mm Hg diastolic before instituting aggressive medical treatment, we believe there is ample evidence for early behavioral and behavioral-pharmacological combined interventions. It is our opinion that waiting this late might result in missing a golden opportunity to more efficiently and naturally control rising blood pressure at a time when the regulatory system (i.e., physiology) is still relatively malleable (Pickering, 1984).

OTHER RISK FACTORS: SMOKING, CHOLESTEROL AND ALCOHOL

We are particularly concerned when one of our hypertensives is also a smoker. As illustrated in our case study, patients should be made keenly aware that the incidence of the most lethal and fastest progressing form of essential hypertension, malignant hypertension (significant 5-year mortality ratio), is much more likely to occur in smokers. In addition to the other behavioral and pharmacological interventions, *smoking treatment should always be strongly recommended*, if not aggressively and directly provided to hypertensives who use tobacco.

Although not emphasized in Chapter 7 on diet and weight, two additional dietary factors have been associated with increased blood pressure and hypertension. Both alcohol (Cooke, Frost & Stokes, 1983) and dietary fat (Puska et al., 1983) have been associated with elevations in blood pressure of 8 mm Hg or more. Although there are some conflicting studies, the Joint National Committee (JNC) on Detection, Evaluation and Treatment of High Blood Pressure (1986) has recommended that (a) serum cholesterol levels be assessed in hypertensives, and, in those for whom it is judged high, restrictions be placed on dietary fat consumption; and (b) in those hypertensives who drink, daily alcohol consumption be reduced to no more than 2 ounces per day, or to abstinence in those showing a BP pressor effect at that drinking level. The JNC, it should be noted, made a particularly strong statement regarding the "compelling and abundant evidence" linking increasing amounts of alcohol ingestion with systematic increases in arterial pressure (JNC, 1986).

ADHERENCE PRECAUTIONS

The possibility of self-management of one's own blood pressure does not come without some risk of problems, however, and clinicians should attend carefully for nonadherence to the behavioral and/or medical intervention and follow-up. Clearly, hypertensives should not be permitted to independently initiate or drop out of treatment without systematic follow-up and, if necessary, medical referral. As indicated earlier, in the absence of adequate training and follow-up, they may believe they are "cured", a disconcertingly common occurrence in our experience.

A FINAL NOTE OF ENCOURAGEMENT

According to the most recent report of the Joint National Committee on Detection, Evaluation and Treatment of High Blood Pressure (1986) more attention should be paid to the nonpharmacologic therapies in the control of hypertension. This volume has not only reviewed the literature in support of the most effective of these approaches, but has also provided a step-by-step approach to implement these programs. As such, we hope this book is found useful by clinical researchers desiring to carefully evaluate the effectiveness of stress management, dietary, and exercise interventions, as well as among clinicians working in a medical setting, or along with physician consultants who want to target the behavioral hypertensive risk factors that may otherwise necessitate a costly, lifetime medication regimen.

References

Acerra, M., Andrasik, F., Blanchard, E. B., Appelbaum, K. A., Fletcher, B., & McCoy, G. C. (1983, March). A comparison of psychological test responses of patients with chronic headache and with essential hypertension. In *Proceedings of the 14th Annual Meeting of the Biofeedback Society of America* (pp. 5–8). Wheat Ridge, CO: Biofeedback Society of America.

Agras, W. S., Schneider, J. A., & Taylor, C. B. (1984). Relaxation training in essential hypertension: A failure of retraining in relaxation procedures. *Behavior Therapy*, **15**, 191–196.

Agras, W. S., Southam, M. A., & Taylor, C. B. (1983). Long-term persistence of relaxation-induced blood pressure lowering during the working day. *Journal of Consulting and Clinical Psychology*, **51**, 792–794.

Agras, W. S., Taylor, C. B., Kraemer, H. C., Allen, R. A., & Schneider, J. A. (1980). Relaxation training: Twenty-four-hour blood pressure reductions. *Archives of General Psychiatry*, **37**, 859–863.

Alderman, H. H., & Schoenbaum, E. E. (1975). Detection and treatment of hypertension at the work site. *New England Journal of Medicine*, **293**, 65–68.

Alexander, F. (1939). Emotional factors in essential hypertension: Presentation of a tentative hypothesis. *Psychosomatic Medicine*, **1**, 173–179.

Alexander, F. (1950). *Psychosomatic medicine*. New York: Norton.

American College of Sports Medicine (ACSM). (1978). Position statement on the recommended quantity and quality of exercise for developing and maintaining fitness in healthy adults. *Medicine and Science in Sports*, **10**, 7–10.

American College of Sports Medicine. (1980). *Guidelines for Graded Exercise Testing and Exercise Prescription*. Philadelphia: Lea & Febiger.

Andrasik, F., Blanchard, E. B., Neff, D. F., & Rodichok, L. D. (1984). Biofeedback and relaxation training for chronic headache: A controlled comparison of booster treatments and regular contacts for long-term maintenance. *Journal of Consulting and Clinical Psychology*, **52**, 609–615.

Andrasik, F., Pallmeyer, T. P., Blanchard, E. B., & Attanasio, V. (1984). Continuous versus interrupted schedules of thermal biofeedback: An exploratory analysis with clinical subjects. *Biofeedback and Self-Regulation*, **9**, 291–298.

Andrew, G. M., Oldridge, N. B., Parker, J. O., Cunningham, D. A., Rechnitzer, P. A., Jones, N. L., Buck, C., Kavanagh, T., Shepard, R. J., Sutton, J. R., & McDonald, W. (1981). Reasons for dropout from exercise programs in post-coronary patients. *Medicine and Science in Sports and Exercise*, **13**, 164–168.

Barry, A., Daly, I., Pruette, E., Steinmetz, J. R., Page, H. F., Birkhead, N. C., & Rodal, K. (1966). The effects of physical conditioning on older individuals. *Journal of Gerontology*, **21**, 182–191.

Beck, A. T., Ward, C. H., Mendelson, M., Mock, J. & Erbaugh, J. (1961). An inventory for measuring depression. *Archives of General Psychiatry*, **5**, 561–571.

Becker, M. H. (1985). Patient adherence to prescribed therapies. *Medical Care*, **23**, 539–555.

Benson, H. (1975). *The relaxation response*. New York: Morrow.

Benson, H. (1977). Systemic hypertension and the relaxation response. *New England Journal of Medicine*, **296**, 1152–1156.

Benson, H., Rosner, B. A., & Marzetta, B. R. (1973). Decreased systolic blood pressure in hypertensive subjects who practiced meditation. *Journal of Clinical Investigation*, **52**, 8.

Benson, H., Rosner, B. A., Marzetta, B. R., & Klemchuk, H. P. (1974a). Decreased blood pressure in borderline hypertensive subjects who practiced meditation. *Journal of Chronic Diseases*, **27**, 163–169.

Benson, H., Rosner, B. A., Marzetta, B. R., & Klemchuk, H. M. (1974b). Decreased blood pressure in pharmacologically treated hypertensive patients who regularly elicited the relaxation response. *Lancet*, **1**, 289–291.

Benson, H., Shapiro, D., Tursky, B., & Schwartz, G. E. (1971). Decreased systolic blood pressure through operant conditioning techniques in patients with essential hypertension. *Science*, **173**, 740–742.

Berchtold, P., Jorgens, V., Kemmer, F. W., & Berger, M. (1982). Obesity and hypertension: Cardiovascular response to weight reduction. *Hypertension*, **4**(Suppl. III), 50–55.

Bernstein, D. A., & Borkovec, T. D. (1973). *Progressive relaxation training*. Champaign, IL: Research Press.

Biron, P., Mongeau, J., & Bertrand, C. (1976). Familiar aggregation of blood pressure in 558 adopted children. *Canadian Medical Association Journal*, **115**, 773–790.

Blackwell, B., Bloomfield, S., Gartside, P., Robinson, A., Hanenson, I., Magenheim, H., Nidich, S., & Zigler, R. (1976). Transcendental meditation in hypertension: Individual response patterns, *Lancet*, 223–226.

Blair, S. N., Goodyear, N. N., Gibbons, L. W., & Cooper, K. H. (1984). Physical fitness and incidence of hypertension in healthy normotensive men and women. *Journal of the American Medical Association*, **252**, 487–490.

Blanchard, E. B., & Andrasik, F. (1982). Psychological assessment and treatment of headache: Recent developments and emerging issues. *Journal of Consulting and Clinical Psychology*, **50**, 859–879.

Blanchard, E. B., & Andrasik, F. (1985). *Management of chronic headache: A psychological approach*. Elmsford, NY: Pergamon Press.

Blanchard, E. B., & Andrasik, F. (1987). Biofeedback treatment of vascular headache. In J. P. Hatch, J. D. Rugh, & J. G. Fisher (Eds.), *Biofeedback Studies in Clinical Efficacy*. NY: Plenum.

Blanchard, E. B., Andrasik, F., Appelbaum, K. A., Evans, D. D., Jurish, S. E., Teders, S. J., Rodichok, L. D., & Barron, K. D. (1985). The efficacy and cost-effectiveness of minimal-therapist-contact, non-drug treatments of chronic migraine and tension headache. *Headache*, **25**, 214–220.

Blanchard, E. B., & Epstein, L. H. (1978). *A biofeedback primer*, Reading, MA: Addison-Wesley.

Blanchard, E. B., McCoy, G. C., Andrasik, F., Acerra, M., Pallmeyer, T. P., Gerardi, R., Halpern, M., & Musso, A. (1984). Preliminary results from a controlled evaluation of thermal biofeedback as a treatment for essential hypertension. *Biofeedback and Self-Regulation*, **4**, 471–495.

Blanchard, E. B., McCoy, G. C., McCaffrey, R. J., Berger, M., Musso, A. J., Wittrock, D. A., Gerardi, M. A., & Halpern, M. (in press). Evaluation of a minimal-therapist-contact thermal biofeedback treatment program for essential hypertension. *Biofeedback and Self-Regulation*.

Blanchard, E. B., McCoy, G. C., McCaffrey, R. J., Wittrock, D. A., Musso, A., Berger, M., Pangburn, L., & Khramelashvili, V. V. (1987, March). *The USSR-USA collaborative cross-cultural comparison of autogenic training and thermal biofeedback in the treatment of mild hypertension*. Presented at Society of Behavioral Medicine. Washington, D.C.

Blanchard, E. B., McCoy, G. C. Musso, A., Gerardi, M. A., Pallmeyer, T. P., Gerardi, R. J., Cotch, P. A., Siracusa, K., & Andrasik, F. (1986). A controlled comparison of thermal biofeedback and relaxation training in the treatment of essential hypertension: I. Short-term and long-term outcome. *Behavior Therapy*, **17**, 563–579.

Blanchard, E. B., Miller, S. T., Abel, G. G., Haynes, M. R., & Wicker, R. (1979). Evaluation of biofeedback in the treatment of borderline essential hypertension. *Journal of Applied Behavior Analysis*, **12**, 99–109.

Blanchard, E. B., Murphy, W. D., Haynes, M. R., & Abel, G. G. (1979, December). *A controlled comparison of four kinds of relaxation training in the treatment of hypertension*. Paper presented at the meeting of Association for Advancement of Behavior Therapy, San Francisco.

Blanchard, E. B., Young, L. D., & Haynes, M. R. (1975). A simple feedback system for the treatment of elevated blood pressure. *Behavior Therapy*, **6**, 241–245.

Bonanno, J. A., & Lies, J. E. (1984). Effects of physical training on coronary risk factors. *American Journal of Cardiology*, **33**, 760–763.

Borg, G. V. (1970). Perceived exertion as indicator of somatic stress. *Scandinavian Journal of Rehabilitative Medicine*, **2**, 92–98.

Borgeat, F., Hade, B., Larouche, L. N., & Bedwani, C. N. (1980). Effects of therapist active presence on EMG biofeedback training of headache patients. *Biofeedback and Self-Regulation*, **5**, 275–282.

Boyer, J. L., & Kasch, F. W. (1970). Exercise therapy in hypertensive men. *Journal of the American Medical Association*, **211**, 1668–1671.

Brandt, E. N. (1983). Assistant Secretary for Health's advisory on treatment of mild hypertension. *FDA Drug Bulletin*, **13**, 24–25.

Brauer, A. B., Horlick, L., Nelson, E., Farquhar, J. W., & Agras, W. S. (1979). Relaxation therapy for essential hypertension: A Veterans Administration outpatient study. *Journal of Behavioral Medicine*, **2**, 21–29.

Breckenridge, A. (1983). Compliance of hypertensive patients with pharmacological treatment. *Hypertension*, **4**(Suppl. III), 85–89.

Brownell, K. D., & Foreyt, J. P. (1985). Obesity. In D. H. Barlow (Ed.), *Clinical handbook of psychological disorders*. New York: Guilford.

Brownell, K. D., & Foreyt, J. P. (1986). *Handbook of eating disorders*. New York: Basic Books.

Budzynski, T. (1978). Biofeedback in the treatment of muscle-contraction (tension) headache. *Biofeedback and Self-Regulation*, **3**, 409–434.

Budzynski, T. H., & Stoyva, J. M. (1969). An instrument for producing deep muscle relaxation by means of analog information feedback. *Journal of Applied Behavior Analysis*, **2**, 231–237.

Budzynski, T., Stoyva, J., & Adler, C. (1970). Feedback-induced muscle relaxation: Application to tension headache. *Journal of Behavior Therapy and Experimental Psychiatry*, **1**, 205–211.

Buss, A. H., & Durkee, A. (1957). An inventory for assessing different kinds of hostility. *Journal of Consulting Psychology*, **21**, 243–248.

Cade, R., Mars, D., Wagemaker, H., Zauner, C., Packer, D., Privette, M., Cade, M.,

Peterson, J., & Hood-Lewis, D. (1984). Effect of aerobic exercise training on patients with systemic arterial tension. *American Journal of Medicine*, **77**, 785–790.

Caggiula, A., Wing, R. R., Nowalk, M. P., Milas, N. C., Lee, S., & Langford, H. (1985). The measurement of sodium and potassium intake. *American Journal of Clinical Nutrition*, **42**, 391–398.

Carnahan, J. E., & Nugent, C. A. (1975). The effects of self-monitoring by patients on the control of hypertension. *American Journal of the Medical Sciences*, **269**, 69–73.

Castelli, W. P. (1984). Epidemiology of coronary heart disease: The Framingham Study. *The American Journal of Medicine*, **76**, 4–12.

Chesney, M. A., Black, G. W., Swan, G. E., & Ward, M. M. (1987). Relaxation training for essential hypertension at the worksite. I: The untreated mild hypertensive. *Psychosomatic Medicine*, **49**, 250–263.

Chiang, B. N., Perlman, L., & Epstein, F. H. (1967). Overweight and hypertension: A review. *Circulation*, **39**, 403–421.

Choquette, G., & Ferguson, R. J. (1973). Blood pressure reduction in "borderline" hypertensives following physical training. *Canadian Medical Association Journal*, **108**, 699–703.

Cochrane, R. (1971). High blood pressure as a psychosomatic disorder: A selective review. *British Journal of Social and Clinical Psychology*, **10**, 61–72.

Cohen, J. D., Grimm, R. H., & Smith, W. M. (1981). Multiple risk factor intervention trial VI: Intervention on blood pressure. *Preventive Medicine*, **10**, 501–518.

Cook, K. M., Frost, G. W., & Stokes, G. S. (1983). Blood pressure and its relationship to low levels of alcohol consumption. *Clinical and Experimental Pharmacology and Physiology*, **10**, 229–244.

Cooper, K. H. (1977). *The aerobics way*. New York: Bantam.

Craig, H. M. (1985). Accuracy of indirect measures of medication compliance in hypertension. *Research in Nursing and Health*, **8**, 61–66.

Dalessio, D. J., Kunzel, M., Sternbach, R., & Slovak, M. (1979). Conditioned adaptation-relaxation reflex in migraine therapy. *Journal of American Medical Association*, **242**, 2102–2104.

Davies, M. H. (1971). Is high blood pressure a psychosomatic disorder? A critical review of the evidence. *Journal of Chronic Disease*, **24**, 239–258.

DeGoulet, P., Menard, J., Vu, H. A., Golmard, J. L., Devries, C., Chatellier, G., & Plouin, P. (1983). Factors predictive of attendance at clinic and blood pressure control in hypertensive patients. *British Medical Journal*, **287**, 88–93.

DePlaen, J. F., & Detry, J. M. (1980). Hemodynamic effects of physical training in established arterial hypertension. *Acta Cardiologica*, **35**, 179–188.

DeQuattro, V., & Miura, Y. (1973). Neurogenic factors in human hypertension: Mechanism or myth? *American Journal of Medicine*, **55**, 362–378.

deVries, H. A. (1970). Physiological effects of an exercise training regimen upon men aged 52 to 88. *Journal of Gerontology*, **25**, 325–340.

Diamond, E. L. (1982). The role of anger and hostility in essential hypertension and coronary heart disease. *Psychological Bulletin*, **92**, 410–433.

DiMatteo, M. R., & DiNicola, D. D. (1982). *Achieving patient compliance: The psychology of the medical practitioner's role*. New York: Pergamon Press.

Dishman, R. K. (1982). Compliance/adherence in health-related exercise. *Health Psychology*, **1**, 237–267.

Dubbert, P. M., Martin, J. E., Zimering, R. T., Burkett, P. A., Lake, M., & Cushman, W. C. (1984). Behavioral control of mild hypertension with aerobic exercise: Two case studies. *Behavior Therapy*, **15**, 373–380.

Dubbert, P. M. (in press). Skinfolds. In M. Hersen & A. S. Bellack (Eds.), *Dictionary of behavioral assessment techniques*. Elmsford, New York: Pergamon Press.

Dubbert, P. M., & Brubaker, R. G. (1987). Assessment of obese patients. In T. D. Nirenberg and S. A. Maisto (Eds.), *Developments in the assessment and treatment of addictive behaviors*. Norwood, NJ: Ablex Publishing Corp, pp. 153–170.

Dubbert, P. M., King, A., Rapp, S., Brief, D., Martin, J. E., & Lake, M. E. (1985). Riboflavin as a tracer of medication compliance. *Journal of Behavioral Medicine*, **8**, 287–289.

Dubbert, P. M., Martin, J. E., & Cushman, W. C. (1985, April). *Medication taste cue contracting for uncontrolled hypertensives*. Presented at the National Conference on High Blood Pressure Control, Chicago.

Dubbert, P. M., & Wilson, G. T. (1983). Failures in behavior therapy for obesity: Causes, correlates, and consequences. In E. Foa & P. M. G. Emmelkamp (Eds.), *Treatment failure in behavior therapy*, New York: Wiley.

Dubbert, P. M., & Wilson, G. T. (1984). Goal-setting and spouse involvement in the treatment of obesity. *Behavior Research and Therapy*, **22**, 227–241.

Dunbar, J. M., Marshall, G. D., & Hovell, M. F. (1979). Behavioral strategies for improving compliance. In R. B. Haynes, D. W. Taylor, & D. L. Sackett (Eds.), *Compliance in health care*. Baltimore: Johns Hopkins University Press.

Dunbar, J. M., & Stunkard, A. J. (1979). Adherence to diet and drug regimen. In R. Levy, B. Rifkind, B. Dennis, & N. Ernst (Eds.), *Nutrition, lipids, and coronary heart disease*. New York: Raven Press.

Duncan. J. J., Farr, J. E., Upton, J., Hagan, R. D., Oglesby, M. E., & Blair, S. N. (1985). The effects of aerobic exercise on plasma catecholamines and blood pressure in patients with mild essential hypertension. *Journal of American Medical Association*, **254**, 2609–2613.

Dustan, H. P. et al. (1958). The effectiveness of long-term treatment of malignant hypertension. *Circulation*, **18**, 644–651.

Elder, S. T., & Eustis, N. K. (1975). Instrumental blood pressure conditioning in out-patient hypertensives. *Behaviour Research & Therapy*, **13**, 185–188.

Elder, S. T., Ruiz, Z. B., Deabler, H. L., & Dillenkoffer, R. L. (1973). Instrumental conditioning of diastolic blood pressure in essential hypertensive patients. *Journal of Applied Behavior analysis*, **6**, 377–382.

Eliahou, H. E., Ianina, A., Gaon, T., Shochat, J., & Modan, M. (1981). Body weight reduction necessary to attain normotension in the overweight hypertensive patient. *International Journal of Obesity*, **5**(Suppl. I), 157–163.

Engel, B. T., Gaarder, K. R., & Glasgow, M. S. (1981). Behavioral treatment of high blood pressure. I. Analyses of intra- and inter-daily variations of blood pressure during a one-month baseline. *Psychosomatic Medicine*, **43**, 255–270.

Engel, B. T., Glasgow, N. S., & Gaardner, K. R. (1983). Behavioral treatment of high blood pressure: III. Follow-up results and treatment recommendations. *Psychosomatic Medicine*, **45**, 23–29.

Epstein, L. H., & Cluss, P. A. (1982). A behavioral medicine perspective on adherence to long-term medical regimens. *Journal of Consulting and Clinical Psychology*, **50**, 950–971.

Eraker, S. A., Kirscht, J. P., & Becker, M. H. (1984). Understanding and improving patient compliance. *Annals of Internal Medicine*, **100**, 258–268.

Eshelman, F. N., & Fitzloff, J. (1976). Effect of packaging on patient compliance with an antihypertensive medication. *Current Therapeutic Research*, **20**, 215–219.

Esler, M., Julius, S., Zweifler, A., Randal, O., Harburg, E., Gardiner, H., & DeQuattro, V. (1977). Mild high-renin hypertension: Neurogenic human hypertension? *New England Journal of Medicine*, **296**, 405–411.

Fahrion, S., Norris, P., Green, A., Green, E., & Snarr, C. (1986). Biobehavioral treatment of essential hypertension: A group outcome study. *Biofeedback and Self-Regulation* **11**, 257–277.

Farquhar, J. W. (1979). *The American way of life need not be hazardous to your health*. New York: W. W. Norton.

Foote, A., & Erfurt, J. C. (1983). Hypertensive control at the work site. *New England Journal of Medicine*, **308**, 809–813.

Freedman, R. R. (1987). Long-term effectiveness of behavioral treatments for Raynaud's Disease. *Behavior Therapy*, **18**, 387–399.

Freis, E. D. (1982). Should mild hypertension be treated? *New England Journal of Medicine*, **307**, 306–309.

Gerardi, R. J., Blanchard, E. B., Andrasik, F., & McCoy, G. C. (1985). Psychological dimensions of "office hypertension." *Behavior Research and Therapy*, **23**, 609–612.

Gillum, R. F., Prineas, R. J., & Elmer, P. J. (1984). Assessing sodium and potassium intake in essential hypertension. *American Heart Journal*, **107**, 549–555.

Glanz, K. (1980). Compliance with dietary regimens: Its magnitude, measurement, and determinants. *Preventive Medicine*, **9**, 787–804.

Glasgow, N. S., Gaardner, K. R., & Engel, B. T. (1982). Behavioral treatment of high blood pressure: II. Acute and sustained effects of relaxation in systolic blood pressure biofeedback. *Psychosomatic Medicine*, **44**, 155–170.

Goldring, W., & Chasis, H. (1965). Anti-hypertensive drug therapy: An appraisal. *Archives of General Psychiatry*, **115**, 523–525.

Goldstein, I. B., Shapiro, D., Thananopavaren, C., & Sambhi, M. P. (1982). Comparison of drug and behavioral treatments of essential hypertension. *Health Psychology*, **1**, 7–26.

Gordis, L. (1979). Conceptual and methodological problems in measuring patient compliance. In R. B. Haynes, D. W. Taylor, & D. L. Sackett (Eds.), *Compliance in health care*. Baltimore: Johns Hopkins University Press.

Green, E. E., Green, A. N., & Norris, P. A. (1979). Preliminary observations on the new non-drug method for control of hypertension. *Journal of the South Carolina Medical Association*, **75**, 575–586.

Guyton, A. C. (1980). *Arterial Pressure and Hypertension*. Philadelphia: Saunders.

Gyntelberg, F. (1974). Physical fitness and coronary heart disease in Copenhagen men aged 40–59. III. Factors related to working capacity. *Danish Medical Bulletin*, **21**, 49–36.

Haber, E. (1985). Hypertension—Where do we go from here? (Editorial) *Hypertension*, **7**, 311–312.

Hagberg, J. M., Goldring, D., Ehsani, A. A., Heath, G. W., Hernandez, A., Schectman, K., & Holloszy, J. O. (1983). Effect of exercise training on the blood pressure and hemodynamic features of hypertensive adolescents. *American Journal of Cardiology*, **52**, 763–768.

Hanson, J. S., & Neede, W. H. (1970). Preliminary observations on physical training for hypertensive males. *Circulation Research*, **27**, 29–57.

Hatch, J. P., Clatt, K. D., Supik, J. D., Rios, N., Fisher, J. G., Bauer, R. L., & Shimotsu, G. W. (1985). Combined behavioral and pharmacological treatment of hypertension. *Biofeedback and Self-Regulation*, **10**, 119–138.

Haynes, R. B. (1979). Introduction. In R. B. Haynes, D. W. Taylor, D. L. Sackett (Eds.), *Compliance in health care*. Baltimore: Johns Hopkins University Press.

Haynes, R. B., Sackett, D. L., Gibson, E. S., Taylor, D. W., Hackett, B. C., Roberts, R. C., & Johnson, A. L. (1976, June). Improvement of medication compliance in uncontrolled hypertension. *Lancet*, 1265–1268.

Haynes, R. B., Taylor, D. W., & Sackett, D. L. (1979). Compliance in health care. Baltimore: Johns Hopkins University Press.

Haynes, R. B., Taylor, D. W., Sackett, D. L., Gibson, S. E., Bernholz, C. D., &

Mukherjee, J. (1980). Can simple clinical measurements detect patient noncompliance? *Hypertension*, **2**, 757–764.

Heide, F. J., & Borkovec, P. D. (1983). Relaxation-induced anxiety: Paradoxical anxiety enchancement due to relaxation training. *Journal of Consulting and Clinical Psychology*, **51**, 171–182.

Hoelscher, T. J. (1987). Maintenance of relaxation-induced blood pressure reductions: Importance of continued relaxation practice. *Biofeedback and Self-Regulation*, **12**, 3–12.

Hoelscher, T. J., Lichstein, K. L., Fischer, S., & Hegarty, T. B. (1987). Relaxation treatment of hypertension: Do home relaxation tapes enhance treatment outcome? *Behavior Therapy*, **18**, 33–37.

Hollandsworth, J. G., Jr. (1986). *Physiology and Behavior Therapy*, New York: Plenum Press.

Holmes, T. H., & Rahe, R. H. (1967). The social readjustment rating scale. *Journal of Psychosomatic Research*, **11**, 213–218.

Holroyd, K. A., Penzien, D. B., Hursey, K. G., Tobin, D. L., Rogers, L., Holm, J. E., Marcille, P. J., Hall, J. R., & Chila, A. G. (1984). Change mechanisms in EMG biofeedback training: Cognitive changes underlying improvements in tension headache. *Journal of Consulting and Clinical Psychology*, **52**, 1039–1053.

Horan, M. J., Blaustein, M. P., Dunbar, J. B., Grundy, S., Kachadorian, W., Kaplan, N. M., Kotchen, T. A., Simopoulos, A. P., & Van Itallie, T. B. (1985). NIH report on research challenges in nutrition and hypertension. *Hypertension*, **7**, 818–823.

Hovell, M. (1986). Chair, Symposium on Hypertension, Society of Behavioral Medicine, San Francisco.

Hovell, M. F. (1982). The experimental evidence for weight-loss treatment of essential hypertension: A critical review. *American Journal of Public Health*, **72**, 359–362.

Hypertension Detection and Follow-up Program Cooperative Group. (1976). The hypertension detection and follow-up program. *Preventive Medicine*, **5**, 207–215.

Hypertension Detection and Follow-up Program Cooperative Group. (1979a). Five-year findings of the hypertension detection and follow-up program. I. Reduction in mortality of persons with high blood pressure, including mild hypertension. *Journal of the American Medical Association*, **242**, 2562–2571.

Hypertension Detection and Follow-up Program Cooperative Group. (1979b). Five-year findings of the hypertension detection and follow-up program. II. Mortality by race, sex and age. *Journal of American Medical Association*, **242**, 2572–2577.

Hypertension Detection and Follow-up Program Cooperation Group. (1982a). Five-year findings of the hypertension detection and follow-up program. III. Reduction and stroke incidence among persons with high blood pressure. *Journal of American Medical Association*, **247**, 633–638.

Hypertension Detection and Follow-up Program Cooperative Group. (1982b). The effect of treatment on mortality and "mild hypertension." *New England Journal of Medicine*, **307**, 976–982.

Jacob, R. G., Kraemer, H. C., & Agras, W. S. (1977). Relaxation therapy in the treatment of hypertension: A review. *Archives of General Psychiatry*, **34**, 1417–1427.

Jacobson, E. (1938). *Progressive relaxation*. Chicago: University of Chicago Press.

James, S. A., Wagner, E. H., Strogatz, D. S., Beresford, S. A. A., Klienbaum, D. G., Williams, C. A., Cutchin, L. M., & Ibrahim, M. A. (1984). The Edgecombe County (NC) high blood pressure control program: II. Barriers to the use of medical care among hypertensive. *American Journal of Public Health*, **74**, 468–471.

Jeffery, R. W., Gillum, R., Gerber, W. M., Jacobs, D., Elmer, P. J., & Prineas, R. J. (1983). Weight and sodium reduction for the prevention of hypertension: A comparison of group treatment and individual counseling. *American Public Health Journal*, **73**, 691–693.

Jenkins, C. D., Zyzanski, S. J., & Rosenman, R. H. (1965). *Jenkins Activity Survey*, New York: Psychological Corporating.

Johnson, W. P., & Grover, J. A. (1967). Hemodynamic and metabolic effects of physical training in four patients with essential hypertension. *Canadian Medical Association Journal*, **96**, 842–845.

Joint National Committee on Detection, Evaluation, and Treatment of High Blood Pressure. (1984). *The 1984 report of the Joint National Committee on Detection, Evaluation, and Treatment of High Blood Pressure* (U.S. Department of Health and Human Services, NIH Publication No. 84–1088). Washington, DC: U.S. Government Printing Office.

Joint National Committee on Detection, Evaluation and Treatment of High Blood Pressure. (1986). Nonpharmacological approaches to the control of high blood pressure. *Hypertension*, **8**, 444–467.

Jurish, S. E., Blanchard, E. B., Andrasik, F., Teders, S. J., Neff, D. F., & Arena, J. G. (1983). Home- versus clinic-based treatment of vascular headache. *Journal of Consulting and Clinical Psychology*, **51**, 743–751.

Kaplan, N. M. (1986). *Clinical hypertension* (4th ed.). Baltimore: Williams & Wilkins.

Kawasaki, T., Delea, C. S., Bartter, F. C., & Smith, H. (1978). The effect of high-sodium and low-sodium intakes on blood pressure and other related variables in human subjects with idiopathic hypertension. *American Journal of Medicine*, **64**, 193–198.

Kentala, E. (1972). Physical fitness and feasibility of physical rehabilitation after mycardial infarction in men of working age. *Annals of Clinical Research*, **4**(Suppl. 9), 1–84.

Kiveloff, B., & Huber, O. (1971). Brief maximal isometric exercise in hypertension. *Journal of the American Geriatric Society*, **19**, 1006–1008.

Kleinert, H. D., Harshfield, G. A., Pickering, T. G., Devereaux, R. B., Sullivan, P. A., Marion, R. M., Malloy, W. K., & Laragh, J. H. (1984). What is the value of home blood pressure measurement in patients with mild hypertension? *Hypertension*, **6**, 574–578.

Kolton, A., & Stone, G. C. (1986). Past and current trends in patient noncompliance research: Focus on diseases, regimens-programs, and provider-disciplines. *The Journal of Compliance in Health Care*, **1**, 21–32.

Kopelman, R. I., & Dzau, V. J. (1985). Trends in the therapy for mild hypertension. A word of caution. *Archives of Internal Medicine*, **145**, 48–49.

Kristt, D. A., & Engel, B. T. (1975). Learned control of blood pressure in patients with high blood pressure. *Circulation*, **51**, 370–378.

Krotkiewski, M., Mandroukas, K., Sjostrom, L., Sullivan, L., Wetterquist, H., & Bjorntorp, P. (1979). Effects of long-term physical training on body fat, metabolism, and blood pressure in obesity. *Metabolism*, **28**, 650–658.

Kukkonen, E., Rauramaa, R., Voutilainen, E., & Lansimies, E. (1982). Physical training of middle-aged men with borderline hypertension. *Annals of Clinical Research*, **14**(Suppl. 34), 139–145.

Langford, H. G. (1982). Drug and dietary intervention in hypertension. *Hypertension*, **4** (Suppl. III), 166–169.

Langford, H. G., Blaufox, D., Oberman, A., Hawkins, M., Curb, J. D., Cutter, G. R., Wassertheil-Smoller, S., Pressel, S., Babcock, C., Abernathy, J. D., Hotchkiss, J., & Tyler, M. (1985). Dietary therapy slows the return of hypertension after stopping prolonged medication. *Journal of the American Medical Association*, **253**, 657–664.

Laragh, J. H., & Pecker, M. S. (1983). Dietary sodium and essential hypertension: Some myths, hopes, and truths. *Annals of Internal Medicine*, **98**, 735–743.

Leon, A. S., Blackburn, H. (1982). Physical activity and hypertension. In E. Fries (Ed.), *Cardiology I. Hypertension*, New York: Butterworth.

Levine, D. M., Green, L. S., Deeds, S. G., Chwalow, J., Russell, R. P., & Finlay, J. (1979). Health education for hypertensive patients. *Journal of the American Medical Association*, **241**, 1700–1703.

Levy, R. I., & Moskowitz, J. (1982). Cardiovascular research: Decades of progress, a decade of promise. *Science*, **217**, 121–129.

Light, K. C., Koepke, J. P., Obrist, P. A., & Willis, P. W. (1983). Psychological stress induces sodium and fluid retention in men at risk for hypertension. *Science*, **220**, 429–431.

Lippold, D. C. J. (1967). Electromyography. In P. H. Venables & I. Martin (Eds.), *Manual of psychophysiological methods*, pp. 245–299. New York: Wiley.

Luft, F. C., Fineberg, N. S., & Sloan, R. S. (1982). Overnight urine collections to estimate sodium intake. *Hypertension*, **4**, 494–498.

Luft, F. C., Sloan, R. S., Fineberg, N. S., & Free, A. H. (1983). The utility of overnight urine collections in assessing compliance with a low sodium intake diet. *Journal of the American Medical Association*, **259**, 1764–1768.

Luft, F. C., Sloan, R. S., Lang, C. L., Cohen, S. J., Fineberg, N. S., Miller, J. Z., & Weinberger, M. H. (1984). Influence of home monitoring on compliance with a reduced sodium diet. *Archives of Internal Medicine*, **144**, 1963–1965.

Luthe, W. (1977). *Introduction to the methods of autogenic therapy*. Wheatridge, CO: The Biofeedback Society of America.

MacGregor, G. A., Markandu, N. D., Best, F. E., Elder, D. M., Cam, J. M., Sagnella, G. A., & Squires, M. (1982). Double-blind randomised crossover trial of moderate sodium restriction in essential hypertension. *Lancet*, **1**, 351–355.

Mahoney, M. J., & Mahoney, K. (1976). *Permanent weight control: A total solution to the dieter's dilemma*. New York: Norton.

Management Committee. (1980). The Australian therapeutic trial in mild hypertension. *Lancet*, 1261–1267.

Mancia, G., Bertini, G., Grassi, G., et al. (1983). Effects of blood pressure measurement by the doctor on patient's blood pressure and heart rate. *Lancet*, **2**, 695–697.

Martin, J. E., Collins, F. L., Jr., Hillenberg, J. B., Zabin, M. A., & Katell, A. D. (1981). Assessing compliance to home relaxation: A simple technology for a critical problem. *Journal of Behavioral Assessment*, **3**, 193–198.

Martin, J. E., & Dubbert, P. M. (1984). Behavioral management strategies for improving health and fitness. *Journal of Cardiac Rehabilitation*, **4**, 200–208.

Martin, J. E., & Dubbert, P. M. (1982). Exercise applications and promotion in behavioral medicine. Current status and future directions. *Journal of Consulting and Clinical Psychology*, **50**, 1004–1017.

Martin, J. E., & Dubbert, P. M. (1985a). Exercise in hypertension. *Annals of Behavioral Medicine*, **7**, 13–18.

Martin, J. E., & Dubbert, P. M. (1985b). Adherence to exercise, In R. J. Terjung (Ed.), *Exercise & Sport Sciences Review*, **13**, 137–167.

Martin, J. E., Dubbert, P. M., Lake, M., & Burkett, P. A. (1982a, November). *The effects of exercise in mild hypertension*. Paper presented before the Annual Convention of the Association for Advancement of Behavior Therapy. Los Angeles, CA.

Martin, J. E., & Dubbert, P. M. (1982b). Exercise and health: The adherence problem. *Behavioral Medicine Update*, **4**, 16–24.

Martin, J. E., Dubbert, P. M., & Cushman, W. C. (1985). Controlled trial of aerobic exercise in hypertension. *Circulation*, **72**, III–13, Suppl. III. (abstract).

Martin, J. E., Dubbert, P. M., & Cushman, W. C. (submitted). Controlled trial of aerobic exercise in hypertension..

Martin, J. E. (1983, November). *Effects of exercise on treatment of hypertension: A controlled study*. National Conference on Non-pharmacological Approaches to Hypertension. Atlantic City, NJ.

Martin, J. E., Dubbert, P. M., Katell, A., Thompson, J. K., Raczynski, J. R., Lake, M., Smith, P. O., Webster, J. S., Sikora, T., & Cohen, R. (1984). The behavioral control of exercise in sedentary adults: Studies 1 through 6. *Journal of Consulting and Clinical Psychology*, **52**, 795–811.

Martin, J. E., Dubbert, P. M., Lake, M., & Burkett, P. (1983). *Effects of exercise on mild hypertension*. Paper presented at the American Public Health Association, Dallas, TX.

McArdle, W. D., Katch, F. I., & Katch, V. L. (1981). *Exercise physiology*. Philadelphia: Lea & Febiger.

McCaffrey, R. J., & Blanchard, E. B. (1985). Stress management approaches to the treatment of essential hypertension. *Annals of Behavioral Medicine*, 7, 5–12.

McCarron, D. A., Morris, C. D., Henry, H. J., & Stanton, J. L. (1984). Blood pressure and nutrient intake in the United States. *Science*, 224, 1392–1398.

McGrady, A. V., Yonker, R., Tan, S. Y., Fine, T. H., & Woerner, M. (1981). The effect of biofeedback-assisted relaxation training on blood pressure and selected biochemical parameters in patients with essential hypertension. *Biofeedback and Self-Regulation*, 6, 353–353.

Miller, N. E. (1972). Postscript. In D. Singh & C. T. Morgan (Eds.), *Current status of physiological psychology: Readings*. Monterey, CA: Brooks-Cole.

Miller, N. E. (1975). Clinical applications of biofeedback: Voluntary control of heart rate, rhythm and blood pressure. In H. I. Russek (Ed.), *New Horizons in Cardiovascular Practice*. Baltimore: University Park Press. (pp. 239–249).

Mohler, E. R., & Freis, E. D. (1960). Five-year survival of patients with malignant hypertension treated with anti-hypertensive agents. *American Heart Journal*, 60, 329–335.

Montoye, H. D. (1978). *An introduction to measurement in physical education*. Boston: Allyn & Bacon.

Montoye, H. J., Metzner, H. L., Keller, J. B., Johnson, B. D., & Epstein, F. H. (1972). Habitual physical activity and blood pressure. *Medical Science in Sports*, 4, 175–181.

Morgan, T., Admam, W., Gillies, A., Wilson, M., Morgan, G., & Carney, S. (1978). Hypertension treated by salt restriction. *Lancet*, 1, 227–230.

Morisky, D. E. (1986). Nonadherence to medical recommendations for hypertensive patients: Problems and potential solutions. *Journal of Compliance in Health Care*, 1, 5–20.

Morisky, D. E., Levine, D. M., Green, L. W., Shapiro, S., Russell, R. P., & Smith, C. R. (1983). Five-year blood pressure control and mortality following health education for hypertensive patients. *American Journal of Public Health*, 73, 153–162.

Morris, J. N., & Crawford, M. D. (1958). Coronary heart disease and physical activity of work. *British Medical Journal*, 2, 1485–1496.

Multiple Risk Factor Intervention Trial Research Group. (1982). Multiple risk factor intervention trial: Risk factor changes in mortality results. *Journal of American Medical Association*, 248, 1465–1477.

National Heart, Lung, and Blood Institute Working Group (1982). Management of patient compliance in the treatment of hypertension. *Hypertension*, 4, 415–423.

Nelson, E. C., Stason, W. B., Neutra, R. R., Solomon, H. S., & McArdle, P. J. (1978). Impact of patient perceptions on compliance with treatment for hypertension. *Medical Care*, 16, 893–906.

Nessman, D. G., Carnahan, J. E., & Nugent, C. A. (1980). Increasing compliance. Patient operated hypertension groups. *Archives of Internal Medicine*, 140, 1427–1430.

Nomura, G., Kumagai, E., Midorikawa, K., Kitano, T. Tashiro, H., & Toshima, H. (1984). Physical training in essential hypertension: Alone and in combination with dietary salt restriction. *Journal of Cardiac Rehabilitation*, 4, 467–475.

Nowalk, M. P., & Wing, R. R. (1985). Changes in nutrient intake of hypertensives during a behavioral weight-control program. *Addictive Behaviors*, 10, 357–363.

Oldridge, N. B. (1982). Compliance and exercise in primary and secondary prevention of coronary heart disease: A review. *Preventive Medicine*, 11, 56–70.

Ost, L. G., & Gotestam, K. G. (1986). Behavioral and pharmacological treatments for obesity: An experimental comparison. *Addictive Behaviors*, 1, 331–338.

Paffenbarger, R. S., Wing, A. L., Hyde, R. T., & Jung, D. L. (1983). Physical activity as an index of hypertension in college alumni. *American Journal of Epidemiology*, **117**, 245–257.

Page, L. B. (1983). Epidemiology of hypertension. In J. Genest. O. Kuchel, P. Hamet, & M. Cantin (Eds.), *Hypertension* (2nd ed.). New York: McGraw-Hill.

Patel, C. H. (1973). Yoga and biofeedback in the management of hypertension. *Lancet*, **2**, 1053–1055.

Patel, C. H. (1977). Biofeedback-aided relaxation and meditation in the management of hypertension. *Biofeedback and Self-Regulation*, **2**, 1–42.

Paul, G. L. (1966). *Insight vs densensitization in psychotherapy: An experiment in anxiety reduction*. Stanford, CA: Stanford University Press.

Paul, G. L., & Trimble, R. W. (1970). Recorded versus "live" relaxation training and hypnotic suggestion: Comparative effectiveness for reducing physiological arousal and inhibiting stress response. *Behavior Therapy*, **1**, 285–302.

Peck, C. L., & King, N. J. (1982). Increasing patient compliance with prescriptions. *Journal of the American Medical Association*, **248**, 2874–2877.

Perera, G. A. (1960). Anti-hypertensive drugs versus symptomatic treatment in primary hypertension: Effect on survival. *Journal of American Medical Association*, **173**, 11–13.

Perloff, D., Sokolow, M., & Cowan, R. (1983). The prognostic value of ambulatory blood pressures. *Journal of American Medical Association*, **249**, 2792–2798.

Peters, R. K., Benson, H., & Peters, J. M. (1977). Daily relaxation response breaks in a working population: II. Effect on blood pressure. *American Journal of Public Health*, **67**, 954–959.

Pickering, G. (1984). *Hypertension: Causes, consequences and management*. London: Churchill Livingstone.

Pickering, T. G., Harshfield, G. A., Devereux, R. B., & Laragh, J. H. (1985). What is the role of ambulatory blood pressure monitoring in the management of hypertension patients? *Hypertension*, **7**, 171–177.

Pickering, T. G., Harshfield, G. A., Kleinert, H. D., Blank, S., & Laragh, J. H. (1982). Blood pressure during normal daily activities, sleep, and exercise: Comparison of values in normal and hypertensive subjects. *Journal of American Medical Association*, **247**, 992–996.

Pikoff, H. (1984). A critical review of Autogenic Training in America. *Clinical Psychology Review*, **4**, 619–639.

Pollack, A. A., Weber, M. A., Case, D. B., & Laragh, J. H. (1977). Limitations of Transcendental Meditation in the treatment of essential hypertension. *Lancet*, 71–73.

Pollock, M. L., Wilmore, J. H., & Fox, S. M., III. (1984). *Exercise in health and disease*. Philadelphia: Saunders.

Prineas, R. J., & Gillum, R. (1985). U.S. Epidemiology of hypertension in blacks. In W. D. Hall, E. Saunders, & N. B. Shulman (Eds.), *Hypertension in blacks*. Chicago: Year Book Medical Publishers.

Puska, P., Iacono, J. M., Nissinen, A., Vartianinen, E., Pietinen, P., Doughery R., Leino, V., Mutanen, M., Moisio, S., & Huttunen, J. (1983). Controlled, randomized trial of the effect of dietary fat on blood pressure. *Lancet*, **1**, 1–5.

Reisin, E., Abel, R., Modan, M., Silverberg, D. S., Eliahou, H., & Modan, B. (1978). Effect of weight loss without salt restriction on the reduction of blood pressure in overweight hypertensive patients. *New England Journal of Medicine*, **298**, 1–5.

Relman, A. S. (1966). In F. J. Ingelfinger, A. S. Relman, & M. Finland (Eds.), *Controversy in Internal Medicine*, (pp. 101–102). Philadelphia: Saunders.

Ressl, J., Chrastek, J., & Jandova, R. (1977). Hemodynamic effects of physical training in essential hypertension. *Acta Cardiologica*, **32**, 121–133.

Richards, A. M., Nicholls, M. G., Espiner, E. A., Ikram, H., Maslowski, A. H., Hamilton,

E. J., & Wells, J. E. (1984). Blood pressure response to moderate sodium restriction and to potassium supplementation in mild hypertension. *Lancet*, **1**, 757–761.

Roman, O., Camuzzi, A. L., Villalon, E., & Klenner, C. (1981). Physical training program in arterial hypertension. A long-term prospective follow-up. *Cardiology*, **67**, 230–243.

Rudd, J. L., & Day, W. D. (1967). A physical fitness program for patients with hypertension. *Journal of Geriatric Society*, **15**, 373–379.

Sackett, D. L. (1979). A compliance practicum for the busy practitioner. In R. B. Haynes, D. W. Taylor, & D. L. Sackett (Eds.), *Compliance in health care*. Baltimore: Johns Hopkins University Press.

Sackett, D. L., Haynes, R. B., Gibson, E. S., Hackett, B. C., Taylor, D. W., Roberts, R. S., & Johnson, A. L. (1975, May). Randomized clinical trial of strategies for improving medication compliance in primary hypertension. *Lancet*, 1205–1207.

Sannerstedt, R., Wasir, H., Henning, R., & Werkö, L. (1973). Systematic hemodynamics in mild arterial hypertension before and after physical training. *Clinical Science and Molecular Medicine*, **45**, 145s–149s.

Schilling, D., & Poppen, R. (1983). Behavioral relaxation training and assessment. *Journal of Behavior Therapy and Experimental Psychiatry*, **14**, 99–107.

Schlundt, D. G. & Langford, H. G. (1985). Dietary approaches to the treatment of hypertension. *Annals of Behavioral Medicine*, **7**, 19–24.

Schultz, J. H., & Luthe, U. (1969). *Autogenic training, vol. I*. New York: Grune & Stratton.

Schwartz, G. E., & Shapiro, D. (1973). Biofeedback and essential hypertension: Current findings and theoretical concerns. In L. Birk (Ed.), *Biofeedback: Behavioral Medicine*. New York: Grune & Stratton.

Seer, P., & Raeburn, J. N. (1980). Meditation training and essential hypertension: A methodological study. *Journal of Behavioral Medicine*, **3**, 59–71.

Shapiro, D. (1974). Operant-feedback control of human blood pressure: Some clinical issues. In P. A. Obrist, A. H. Black, J. Brener, & L. V. DiCara (Eds.), *Cardiovascular Psychophysiology*. Chicago: Aldine.

Shapiro, D., Tursky, B., & Schwartz, G. E. (1970). Control of blood pressure in man by operant conditioning. *Circulation Research*, **26**(Suppl. 1), 27–32.

Shapiro, D., Tursky, B., Gershon, E., & Stern, M. (1969). Effects of feedback and reinforcement on control of human systolic blood pressure. *Science*, **163**, 588–590.

Shapiro, D. (1977). A monologue on biofeedback in psychophysiology. *Psychophysiology*, **14**, 213–227.

Shaw, E. R., & Blanchard, E. B. (1983). The effects of instructional set on the outcome of a stress management program. *Biofeedback and Self-Regulation*, **8**, 555–565.

Sims, E. A. H. (1982). Mechanisms of hypertension in the overweight. *Hypertension*, **4** (Suppl. III). 43–49.

Sokolow, M., & Perloff, D. (1960). Five-year survival of consecutive patients with malignant hypertension treated with anti-hypertensive agents. *American Journal of Cardiology*, **6**, 858–863.

Southam, M. A., Agras, W. S., Taylor, C. B., & Kramer, H. C. (1982). Relaxation training: Blood pressure lowering during the working day. *Archives of General Psychiatry*, **39**, 715–717.

Spielberger, C. D. (1980). *Preliminary manual for the State-Trait Anger Scale (STAS)*. Tampa, FL: Center for Research in Community Psychology, University of South Florida.

Spielberger, C. D., Gorsuch, R. L., & Luschene, R. E. (1970). *STAI manual for the State-Trait Anxiety Inventory*. Palo Alto, CA: Consulting Psychologists Press.

Stamler, J., Farinaro, E., Mojonnier, L. M., Hall, Y., Moss, D. E., & Stamler, R. (1980). Prevention and control of hypertension by nutritional-hygienic means. *Journal of the American Medical Association*, **243**, 1819–1823.

Steckel, S. B., & Swain, M. A. (1977). Contracting with patients to improve compliance. *Hospitals*, **51**, 81–84.

Steiner, S. S., & Dince, W. N. (1981). Biofeedback efficacy studies: A critique of critiques. *Biofeedback and Self-Regulation*, **6**, 275–288.

Steinhaus, A. H. (1933). Chronic effects of exercise. *Physiological Review*, **12**, 103–147.

Stone, R. A., & DeLeo, J. (1976). Psychotherapeutic control of hypertension. *New England Journal of Medicine*, **294**, 80–84.

Stoyva, J., & Budzynski, T. (1974). Cultivated low arousal—An antistress response? In L. V. DiCara (Ed.), *Limbic and autonomic nervous systems research*. New York: Plenum.

Stuart, R. B., & Davis, B. (1972). *Slim chance in a fat world*. Champaign, IL: Research Press.

Stunkard, A. J., Wilcoxon-Craighead, L., & O'Brien, R. (1980). Controlled trial of behavior therapy, pharmacotherapy, and their combination in the treatment of obesity. *Lancet*, **1**, 1045–1047.

Subcommittee on Definition and Prevalence of the 1984 Joint National Committee. (1985). Hypertension prevalence and the status of awareness, treatment, and control in the United States. *Hypertension*, **7**, 457–468.

Subcommittee on Nonpharmacological Therapy of the 1984 Joint National Committee. (1986). Nonpharmacological approaches to the control of high blood pressure. *Hypertension*, **8**, 444–467.

Surwit, R. S., & Keefe, F. J. (1978). Frontalis EMG feedback training: An electronic panacea? *Behavior Therapy*, **9**, 779–792.

Surwit, R. S., Shapiro, D., & Good, I. M. (1978). Comparison of cardiovascular biofeedback, neuromuscular biofeedback, and meditation in the treatment of borderline essential hypertension. *Journal of Consulting and Clinical Psychology*, **46**, 252–263.

Surwit, R. S., Williams, R. B., & Shapiro, D. (1982). *Behavioral approaches to cardiovascular disease*, New York: Academic Press.

Swain, M. A., & Steckel, S. B. (1981). Influencing adherence among hypertensives. *Research in Nursing and Health*, **4**, 213–222.

Takala, J., Niemela, N., Posti, J., & Sievers, K. (1979). Improving compliance with therapeutic regimens in hypertensive patients in a community health center. *Circulation*, **59**, 540–543.

Taub, E., & School, P. J. (1978). Some methodological considerations in thermal biofeedback training. *Behavioral Research Methods and Instrumention*, **10**, 617–622.

Taylor, C. B., Agras, W. S., Schneider, J. A., & Allen, R. A. (1983). Adherence to instructions to practice relaxation exercises. *Journal of Consulting and Clinical Psychology*, **51**, 952–953.

Taylor, C. B., Farquhar, J. W., Nelson, E., & Agras, W. S. (1977). Relaxation therapy and high blood pressure. *Archives of General Psychiatry*, **34**, 339–343.

Thompson, J. K., & Martin, J. E. (1984). Exercise in health modification: Assessment and training guidelines. *Behavior Therapist*, **7**, 5–8.

Tipton, C. M. (1984). Exercise training and hypertension. *Exercise and Sport Science Reviews*, **12**, 245–306.

Tuck, M. L., Sowers, J., Dornfeld, L., Kledzik, G., & Maxwell, M. (1981). The effect of weight reduction on blood pressure, plasma renin activity, and plasma aldosterone levels in obese patients. *New England Journal of Medicine*, **304**, 930–933.

Veterans Administration Cooperative Study Group on Antihypertensive Agents. (1967). Effects of treatment morbidity in hypertension: Results in patients with diastolic blood pressures averaging 115 through 129 mm Hg. *Journal of American Medical Association*, **202**, 1028–1034.

Veterans Administration Cooperative Study Group on Antihypertensive Agents. (1970). Effects of treatment on morbidity in hypertension: II. Results in patients with diastolic blood pressure averaging 90 through 114 mm Hg. *Journal of American Medical Association*, **213**, 1142–1152.

Wadden, T. A., & Stunkard, A. J. (1986). Controlled trial of very low calorie diet, behavior therapy, and their combination in the treatment of obesity. *Journal of Consulting and Clinical Psychology*, **54**, 482–488.

Wadden, T. A., Stunkard, A. J., & Brownell, K. D. (1983). Very low calorie diets: Their efficacy, safety, and future, *Annals of Internal Medicine*, **99**, 675–684.

Wagner, E. H., Truesdale, R. A., & Warner, J. T. (1981). Compliance, treatment practices, and blood pressure control: Community survey findings. *Journal of Chronic Disease*, **34**, 519–525.

Watts, R. J. (1981). Sexual functioning, health beliefs, and compliance with high blood pressure medication. *Nursing Research*, **31**, 278–283.

Weder, A. B., & Julius, S. (1985). Behavior, blood pressure variability, and hypertension. *Psychosomatic Medicine*, **47**, 406–414.

Weiner, H. (1977). *Psychobiology and human disease*. New York: Elsevier.

Whitehead, W. E., Blackwell, B., DeSilva, H., & Robinson, A. (1977). Anxiety and anger in hypertension. *Journal of Psychosomatic Research*, **21**, 383–389.

Widmer, R. B., Cadoret, R. J., & Troughton, E. (1983). Compliance characteristics of 291 hypertensive patients from a rural midwest area. *Journal of Family Practice*, **17**, 619–625.

Williams, C. A., Beresford, S. A. A., James, S. A., LaCroix, A. Z., Strogaz, D. S., Wagner, E. H., Kleinbaum, D. C., Cutchin, L. M., & Ibrahim, M. A. (1985). The Edgecombe County high blood pressure control program: III. Social support, social stressors, and treatment dropout. *American Journal of Public Health*, 483–486.

Wilmore, J. H., Royce, J., Girandola, R. N., Katch, F. I., & Katch, V. L. (1970). Physiological alterations resulting from a 10-week program of jogging. *Medical Science in Sports*, **2**, 7–14.

Wing, R. R., Caggiula, A. W., Nowalk, M. P., Koeske, R., Lee, S., & Langford, H. (1984). Dietary approaches to the reduction of blood pressure: The independence of weight and sodium/potassium interventions. *Preventive Medicine*, **13**, 233–244.

Wolpe, J. (1958). *Psychotherapy by reciprocal inhibition*. Stanford, CA: Stanford University Press.

Working Group on Risk and High Blood Pressure. (1985). An epidemological approach to describing risk associated with blood pressure levels. *Hypertension*, **7**, 641–651.

Zismer, D. K., Gillum, R. F., Johnson, C. A., Becerra, J., & Johnson, T. H. (1982). Improving hypertension control in a private medical practice. *Archives of Internal Medicine*, **142**, 297–299.

Author Index

Subject Index

About the Authors

EDWARD B. BLANCHARD, Ph.D.

Ed Blanchard received his Ph.D. in clinical psychology from Stanford University in 1969. He subsequently was on the faculty at the University of Georgia, University of Mississippi Medical Center, and University of Tennessee Center for the Health Sciences. Since 1977, he has been Professor of Psychology at SUNY-Albany. He has been President of the Health Psychology Division (Division 38) of the American Psychological Association and Editor of both *Behavior Therapy* and *Biofeedback and Self-Regulation*. His work with biofeedback and cardiovascular responses began in 1970. Since 1973 he has been engaged in research and clinical practice involving various biofeedback and relaxation treatments for hypertension.

JOHN E. MARTIN, Ph.D.

John Martin received his Ph.D. in clinical psychology from Auburn University in 1978. He served on the faculty at the V.A. Medical Center and University of Mississippi Medical Center in Jackson, Miss., with appointments in psychology, psychiatry and medicine, from 1978 to 1986. In 1986 he accepted a position as Professor and Co-Director of the Joint Doctoral Program in Clinical Psychology at San Diego State University (in conjunction with University of California, San Diego, School of Medicine). He has been Associate Editor of *Journal of Applied Behavior Analysis*, and Consulting Editor for *Behavioral Medicine Abstracts*. He has been conducting research on the behavioral control of high blood pressure and exercise since 1979.

PATRICIA M. DUBBERT, Ph.D.

Pat Dubbert received her M.A. in psychiatric-mental health nursing from New York University in 1972 and her Ph.D. in clinical psychology from Rutgers University in 1982. She has worked as a clinical nurse specialist, a member of the nursing faculty at Herbert Lehman College of the City University of New York, and a consultant to the Live for Life Program at Johnson & Johnson. Subsequent to completing psychology residency training at the University of Mississippi and Jackson VA Medical Centers in 1981, she served as project director of the Cardiovascular Risk Modification Program and staff psychologist at the Jackson VA Medical Center. Currently, she is Chief of the Psychology Service at the Jackson VA Medical Center and Associate Professor of Psychiatry and Human Behavior (Psychology) at the University of Mississippi Medical Center.

Psychology Practitioner Guidebooks

Editors
Arnold P. Goldstein, Syracuse University
Leonard Krasner, Stanford University & SUNY at Stony Brook
Sol L. Garfield, Washington University

Elsie M. Pinkston & Nathan L. Linsk—CARE OF THE ELDERLY: A Family Approach

Donald Meichenbaum—STRESS INOCULATION TRAINING

Sebastiano Santostefano—COGNITIVE CONTROL THERAPY WITH CHILDREN AND ADOLESCENTS

Lillie Weiss, Melanie Katzman & Sharlene Wolchik—TREATING BULIMIA: A Psychoeducational Approach

Edward B. Blanchard & Frank Andrasik—MANAGEMENT OF CHRONIC HEADACHES: A Psychological Approach

Raymond G. Romanczyk—CLINICAL UTILIZATION OF MICROCOMPUTER TECHNOLOGY

Philip H. Bornstein & Marcy T. Bornstein—MARITAL THERAPY: A Behavioral-Communications Approach

Michael T. Nietzel & Ronald C. Dillehay—PSYCHOLOGICAL CONSULTATION IN THE COURTROOM

Elizabeth B. Yost, Larry E. Beutler, M. Anne Corbishley & James R. Allender—GROUP COGNITIVE THERAPY: A Treatment Method for Depressed Older Adults

Lillie Weiss—DREAM ANALYSIS IN PSYCHOTHERAPY

Edward A. Kirby & Liam K. Grimley—UNDERSTANDING AND TREATING ATTENTION DEFICIT DISORDER

Jon Eisenson—LANGUAGE AND SPEECH DISORDERS IN CHILDREN

Eva L. Feindler & Randolph B. Ecton—ADOLESCENT ANGER CONTROL: Cognitive-Behavioral Techniques

Michael C. Roberts—PEDIATRIC PSYCHOLOGY: Psychological Interventions and Strategies for Pediatric Problems

Daniel S. Kirschenbaum, William G. Johnson & Peter M. Stalonas, Jr.—TREATING CHILDHOOD AND ADOLESCENT OBESITY

W. Stewart Agras—EATING DISORDERS: Management of Obesity, Bulimia and Anorexia Nervosa

Ian H. Gotlib & Catherine A. Colby—TREATMENT OF DEPRESSION: An Interpersonal Systems Approach

Walter B. Pryzwansky & Robert N. Wendt—PSYCHOLOGY AS A PROFESSION: Foundations of Practice

Cynthia D. Belar, William W. Deardorff & Karen E. Kelly—THE PRACTICE OF CLINICAL HEALTH PSYCHOLOGY

Paul Karoly & Mark P. Jenson—MULTIMETHOD ASSESSMENT OF CHRONIC PAIN

William L. Golden, E. Thomas Dowd & Fred Friedberg—HYPNOTHERAPY: A Modern Approach

Patricia Lacks—BEHAVIORAL TREATMENT FOR PERSISTENT INSOMNIA

Arnold P. Goldstein & Harold Keller—AGGRESSIVE BEHAVIOR: Assessment and Intervention

C. Eugene Walker, Barbara L. Bonner & Keith L. Kaufman—THE PHYSICALLY AND SEXUALLY ABUSED CHILD: Evaluation and Treatment

Robert E. Becker, Richard G. Heimberg & Alan S. Bellack—SOCIAL SKILLS TRAINING TREATMENT FOR DEPRESSION

Richard F. Dangel & Richard A. Polster—TEACHING CHILD MANAGEMENT SKILLS

Albert Ellis, John F. McInerney, Raymond DiGiuseppe & Raymond Yeager—RATIONAL-EMOTIVE THERAPY WITH ALCOHOLICS AND SUBSTANCE ABUSERS

Johnny L. Matson & Thomas H. Ollendick—ENHANCING CHILDREN'S SOCIAL SKILLS: Assessment and Training

Edward B. Blanchard, John E. Martin & Patricia M. Dubbert—NON-DRUG TREATMENTS FOR ESSENTIAL HYPERTENSION

Samuel M. Turner & Deborah C. Beidel—TREATING OBSESSIVE-COMPULSIVE DISORDER